Clinical Guide to
ORAL IMPLANTOLOGY
Step by Step Procedures

Clinical Guide to
ORAL IMPLANTOLOGY
Step by Step Procedures

Third Edition

Edited by

Porus S Turner
M.D.S., M.sc. Oral Implantology (Germany)
Professor Emeritus,
Dept. of Prosthodontics & Oral Implantology
A.B. Shetty Institute of Dental Sciences
Nitte University, Mangaluru, Karnataka, India

Ferzin Turner Vazifdar
M.D.S., M.sc. Oral Implantology (Germany)
World Dental Speciality
Mumbai, Maharashtra, India

Ashdin P. Turner
M.D.S., M.sc. Oral Implantology (Germany)
World Dental Speciality
Mumbai, Maharashtra, India

Danesh R. Vazifdar
Adaro Dental Labs.

Foreword
Georg Hubert Nentwig

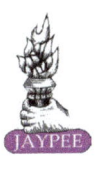

The Health Sciences Publisher
New Delhi | London | Panama

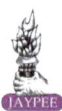
Jaypee Brothers Medical Publishers (P) Ltd

Headquarters
Jaypee Brothers Medical Publishers (P) Ltd
4838/24, Ansari Road, Daryaganj
New Delhi 110 002, India
Phone: +91-11-43574357
Fax: +91-11-43574314
Email: jaypee@jaypeebrothers.com

Overseas Offices

J.P. Medical Ltd
83 Victoria Street, London
SW1H 0HW (UK)
Phone: +44 20 3170 8910
Fax: +44 (0)20 3008 618
Email: info@jpmedpub.com

Jaypee-Highlights Medical Publishers Inc
City of Knowledge, Bld. 235, 2nd Floor,
Clayton, Panama City, Panama
Phone: +1 507-301-0496
Fax: +1 507-301-0499
Email: cservice@jphmedical.com

Jaypee Brothers Medical Publishers (P) Ltd
17/1-B Babar Road, Block-B, Shyamoli
Mohammadpur, Dhaka-1207
Bangladesh
Mobile: +08801912003485
Email: jaypeedhaka@gmail.com

Jaypee Brothers Medical Publishers (P) Ltd
Bhotahity, Kathmandu, Nepal
Phone: +977-9741283608
Email: kathmandu@jaypeebrothers.com

Website: www.jaypeebrothers.com
Website: www.jaypeedigital.com

© 2018, Jaypee Brothers Medical Publishers

The views and opinions expressed in this book are solely those of the original contributor(s)/author(s) and do not necessarily represent those of editor(s) of the book.

All rights reserved. No part of this publication may be reproduced, stored or transmitted in any form or by any means, electronic, mechanical, photocopying, recording or otherwise, without the prior permission in writing of the publishers.

All brand names and product names used in this book are trade names, service marks, trademarks or registered trademarks of their respective owners. The publisher is not associated with any product or vendor mentioned in this book.

Medical knowledge and practice change constantly. This book is designed to provide accurate, authoritative information about the subject matter in question. However, readers are advised to check the most current information available on procedures included and check information from the manufacturer of each product to be administered, to verify the recommended dose, formula, method and duration of administration, adverse effects and contraindications. It is the responsibility of the practitioner to take all appropriate safety precautions. Neither the publisher nor the author(s)/editor(s) assume any liability for any injury and/or damage to persons or property arising from or related to use of material in this book.

This book is sold on the understanding that the publisher is not engaged in providing professional medical services. If such advice or services are required, the services of a competent medical professional should be sought.

Every effort has been made where necessary to contact holders of copyright to obtain permission to reproduce copyright material. If any have been inadvertently overlooked, the publisher will be pleased to make the necessary arrangements at the first opportunity. The **CD/DVD-ROM** (if any) provided in the sealed envelope with this book is complimentary and free of cost. **Not meant for sale.**

Inquiries for bulk sales may be solicited at: jaypee@jaypeebrothers.com

Clinical Guide to Oral Implantology: Step by Step Procedures

The First and second Editions Published by other Publisher.

Third Edition: **2018**

ISBN 978-93-5270-427-9

Printed at

Foreword

Oral rehabilitation based on implant therapy surpasses all the so called conventional prosthodontic methods which were taught and applied in the past. In fact, an implant can imitate the lost tooth in all ways related to function and esthetics in a perfect way. However, to achieve an excellent result requires a well-educated dental team. Most of the patients today, are well informed about dental implants by the media and become more and more aware and interested in personal health and well-being. They are demanding and expecting best outcomes. Consequently, dentists who want to acquire professional knowledge and skills cannot do this by way of 'learning by doing'. They need from the beginning reliable guidelines provided by professional teachers.

    The presented book is exactly what it is called; 'A clinical guide' to demonstrate and explain the different stages and steps in oral rehabilitation with implants. It is ideal for those who want to get a sound introduction in this field as they will become confronted with all the varieties from simple cases to advanced and complicated ones. Lots of illustrations in excellent quality like in an atlas accompany the presented cases. Besides this, the book is backed up with the right dose of scientific information. Preoperative medical considerations are addressed as well as possible complications which may occur during or after implant therapy.

    This book is not designed to provide the full range of contemporary clinical and academic knowledge on the field of implantology, but it shows a pathway to get the access to it. It is written by a team of enthusiastic and experienced dentists, Implantologists and technicians whom the reader will get great benefit and inspiration from.

Georg Hubert Nentwig, Frankfurt/Germany

The Third Edition is only possible due to
the continuous and generous support from
Colgate Palmolive India Ltd. Their unstinted
support towards continuing dental education
is most gratefully acknowledged.

Preface

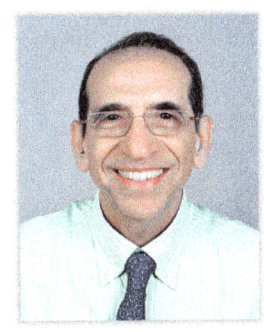

The book is written with the idea of presenting the experience and concepts of the senior author who has been practicing Implant Dentistry since the last 20 years. It is written for the practicing implant dentist as well as for the beginner who wishes to embark upon an implant practice.

Although this book is directed principally for the Ankylos Implant System, first introduced by Prof. Georg Hubert Nentwig and Mr. Moser more than 20 years ago, the principles, and techniques will apply to all implant systems.

It covers not only the standard surgical techniques, but also advances in guided bone regeneration using bone substitutes and membranes. Sinus floor elevation allows rehabilitation even where bone deficiencies exist and has helped numerous patients with the benefit of fixed teeth for function, esthetics and improved quality of life.

Immediate extraction and loading has ceased to be a controversial modality and numerous patients have been rehabilitated faster and better than before.

Long-term preservation of bone and soft tissue surrounding implants has been the goal of implantologists, but till recently not completely achieved. However with the introduction of newer implant systems with progressive threads, growth activating surfaces, and most importantly with conical tapered connections instead of butt joints stability of hard and soft tissues is possible.

The authors with the help of clinical cases will document the treatment planning, surgical steps and rehabilitation in standard sites as also in bone defects to achieve long-term reliability.

The authors wish to particularly thank Prof. Georg Hubert Nentwig who has been a mentor, guide and support to them over the last 10 years. His concepts of implant education, implant surgery, research and innovation have been a guiding beacon for us to follow.

We would also like to thank Nitte Deemed University and in particular its Chancellor Mr. Vinaya Hegde, for his encouragement and for providing facilities without which this publication would not have been possible.

The author is also indebted to the Indian Dental Associations', Secretary General Dr. Ashok Dhoble, for his constant encouragement, support and guidance.

We would also like to acknowledge Dentsply Implants, for their continuing support in the preparation of this treatment guide.

The significant contributions of our associates Bilquis Ghadiali, Farzana Irani, Riddhi Mehta, Radhika Parekh, Cyrus Karkaria, Rushad Nariman and Kaiwan Shroff are most gratefully acknowledged by the authors.

The authors will always remain indebted to Dr. Mehroo P. Turner, for her continuous guidance and support during writing of this book. We would also like to appreciate the excellent support received from Adaro Dental Laboratory in fabrication of the restorations.

Lastly, we would like to thank our composer Mr. Jai Joshi, for his excellent support and to all personnel of Jaypee Brother Medical Publishers (P) Ltd. throughout the preparation of this publication.

Email : porusturner@gmail.com
turnerdents@gmail.com
Website: www.world-dent.com

Contents

Chapter 1. Introduction to Implantology   1
- What is Osseointegration?   2
- Bone Biology, Implant Healing and the Implant Tissue Interphase   5
- Osseointegration   6

Chapter 2. Diagnosis and Treatment Planning   7
- Implant-Retained Fixed Bridges   8
- Implant-Retained Overdentures   10
- Single Tooth Restorations   12
- Planning Considerations   14
- Functional Considerations   14
- Aesthetic Considerations   15
- Study Cast and Diagnostic Set-up   16
- Implant Size, Number and Spacing   19
- Absolute medical Contraindications   19
- Relative Contraindications   19
- Patients on Biphosphonate Therapy   19
- Psychiatric Contraindications   19

Chapter 3. Basic Implant Surgery   21
- Surgical Protocol   21
- Ankylos Implant Site Preparation   24
- Placement of an Ankylos Implant in Standard Posterior Sites: Step-by-step Procedures   26

Chapter 4. Impression Making for Implant Supported Prosthesis   40
- Gingival Health   40
- Impression Technique   41
- Impression making for Implant Dupported Prosthesis   45

Chapter 5. Bone Regeneration   52
- Bone Substitutes   53
- Case 1   54
- Case 2   58
- Case 3   61

Chapter 6. Sinus Grafting   69
- Reconstruction of the Atrophic Posterior Maxilla   69
- Access Window to the Sinus Cavity   74
- Elevation of the Sinus Membrane   76
- Complications   80
- Case Report   81
- Discussion   94

Chapter 7. Crestal Sinus Floor Elevation   95
- Surgical Technique   97
- Case 1   98
- Case 2   101
- Case 3   104

Chapter 8. Immediate Implantation and Provisionalization in the Anterior Maxilla   108
- Crestal Bone Loss and the Biologic Width   108
- Case 1   111
- Case 2   116

Chapter 9. Implant Aesthetics   121
- Case Report   124

Chapter 10. The Ankylos SynCone Concept   134
- Immediately loaded Implant Supported Prosthesis with SynCone   134

Chapter 11. Complete Denture Stabilization Using Two Individual Implants   154
- Case Report   155

Chapter 12. Challenging Implant Cases and Their Management   158
- Case 1   158
- Treatment Plan   159
- Treatment   159
- Discussion   159
- Case 2   161
- Treatment Plan   161
- Treatment   161
- Discussion   163
- Case 3   167
- Discussion   173
- Case 4   174
- Treatment Plan   174
- Treatment   175
- Discussion   175

Chapter 13.	**Complications After Implant Placement**	**179**
	• Case 1 179	
	• Case 2 182	
	• Case 3 184	
Chapter 14.	**Principles of Suturing**	**186**
	• Suturing Instruments 187	
	• Suturing Techniques 189	
	• Surgeon's Knot 195	
Chapter 15.	**Subepithelial Connective Tissue Grafting for Implant Aesthetics**	**199**
	• Modified Tunnel Technique to Thicken Mucosa Around Implants 200	
Chapter 16.	**Maintenance of Implant Rehabilitated Patients**	**205**
	• Importance of Oral Hygiene in Implant Patients 205	
	• Schedule for Maintenance of Implant Patients 207	
	• Abutment Connection 207	
	• Importance of Cessation of Tobacco Habits 207	
Index		*209*

Introduction to Implantology

INTRODUCTION

The goal of implant therapy is to restore an individual to normal anatomy, function, aesthetics, comfort and speech regardless of the loss of bone due to disease or injury to the stomatognathic system. Based on the concepts of osseointegration described by Branemark more than 50 years ago implant dentistry has evolved extensively and has become an integral part in dental rehabilitation.[1] Though it was developed primarily to rehabilitate fully edentulous patients, and it has gradually shifted to partially edentulous patients. Today single tooth replacement by implant has become the number one indication rather than fixed prosthodontics (bridge) because of increased risk of pulpal damage, secondary caries, factures of abutment teeth and periodontal disease (Figs. 1.1A and B). Today implants are no longer placed only in areas where adequate width and height of bone are available but due to the significant advances in bone augmentation procedures implants are placed wherever prosthesis are required.

Guided-bone regeneration with or without membranes and sinus floor elevation have become standards of care to correct bone deficiencies in other parts of the oral cavity. Improved osteophylic microstructured titanium implant surfaces such as the Plus Surface (Dentsply Sirona Implants) significantly

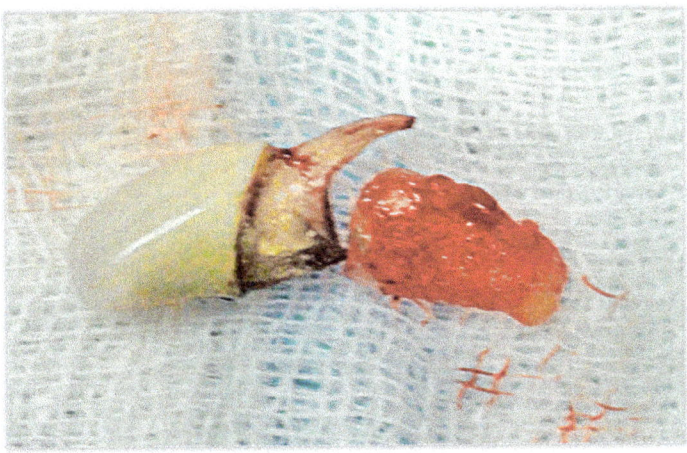

Fig. 1.1A: Horizontal fracture of lateral incisor.

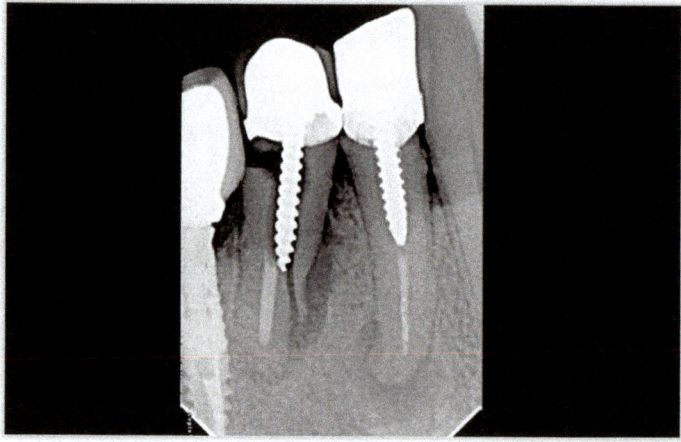

Fig. 1.1B: Radiographic view of vertical fracture of canine.

reduce treatment time because of accelerated growth of bone.[2] These advances in implant therapy have made implants more predictable and attractive to patients. This has also led to more dentists placing implants in daily practice then ever before.

WHAT IS OSSEOINTEGRATION?

Osseointegration refers to incorporation of an inanimate metallic component into living bone. A successful osseointegrated implant is one in which there is a direct connection between ordered living bone and titanium. This attachment must be able to endure conditions of loading. There is no fibrous tissue intervening between the implant and bone, hence the osseointegrated implant is more akin to an ankylosed tooth root. The success of osseointegration has been proven beyond all doubts, however successful achievement of osseointegration depends on careful planning, meticulous surgical technique and skilful prosthetic management. It demands an appreciation of bone biology and wound healing in particular.

The prepared implant site is treated correctly as a wound in which tissue damage has to be minimized. The special characteristics of titanium particularly its resistance to corrosion and its biocompatibility are important. When these above criteria are met living bone recognizes titanium as its own and not as a foreign object.

Types of Dental Implants

Implants may be classified according to their position in the bone, constituent material, and their morphologic design.

Position in the bone

Implants may be subperiosteal, transosseous, or endosseous.

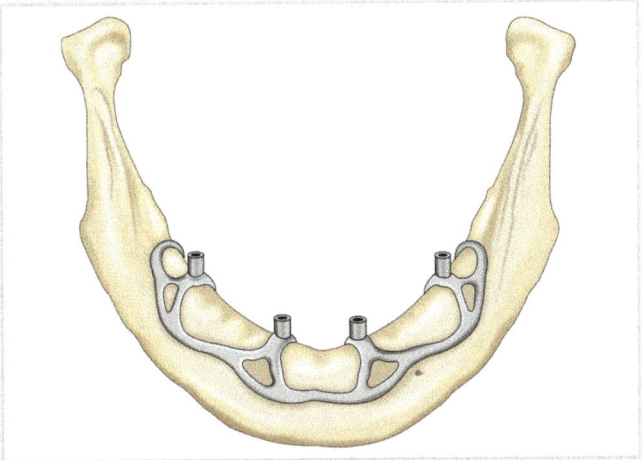

Fig. 1.2: Subperiosteal Implant.

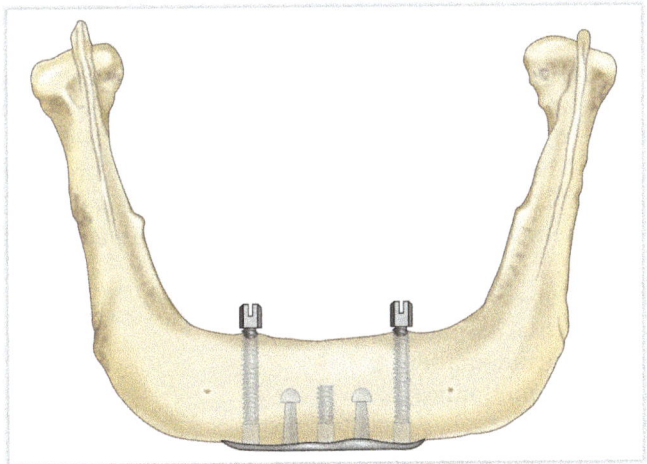

Fig. 1.3: Transosseous Implant.

Subperiosteal Implant

Subperiosteal implant is a non-osseointegrated implant which rests on the surface of the bone below the mucoperiosteum (Fig. 1.2). Some of these implants may have served the patients well for several years but even the best of case reports have not shown success rates over 10 years. Problems have included infection, exposure of framework by down growth of epithelium and damage to the bone. Removal of these implants are also often difficult.

Transosseous Implants

The most common example of a transosseous implant is the mandibular staple implant. It has a plate which fits on to the lower border of the mandible at the symphysis and has posts arising from it (Fig. 1.3). Some of these posts pass into the jaws and others pass transosseously into the mouth where they serve to stabilize a denture. They are used only in the mandible. Bone loss around the post has been a common problem.

Endosseous Implants

Endosseous implants are placed into the maxilla or mandible from intraoral incisions after raising the mucoperiosteum and drilling into the bone. The shapes and construction materials vary, however the most common today is a tapered microtextured screw implant (Fig. 1.4). They may be used to replace single teeth, partially edentulous jaws or totally edentulous jaws. Most claim to be osseointegrated.

Materials

The most frequently used material for dental implants today is pure titanium or a titanium alloy. However, Zirconia implants are also available commercially.

Designs

There are numerous implant designs in the market, however the most prevalent today is the solid screw, which confirms to the shape of the tooth root and has a microtextured rough surface. An example of a good design is the Ankylos C/X Implant, Xive (Dentsply Sirona Implants), Noble Implant System and Straumann Implant System. In a survey of practicing dentists, Worthington listed the following features as important in making a right choice for an implant system:
- Demonstration of reliability (over at least 5 years)
- American Dental Association Approval
- Quality of instrumentation
- Quality of Prosthodontics
- Versatility
- Reputation of the manufacturing company

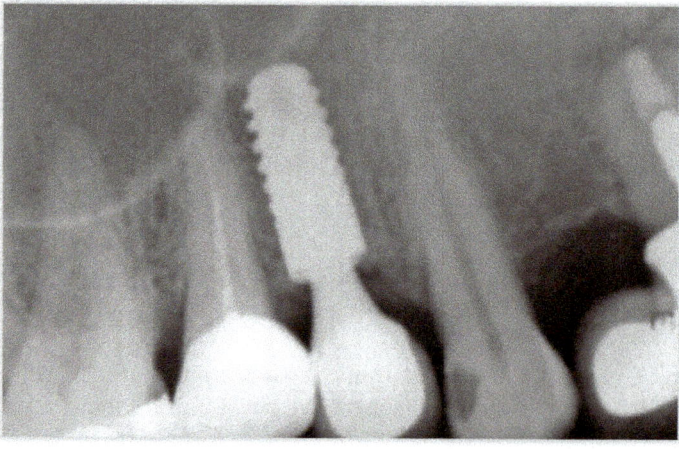

Fig. 1.4: Endosseous Implant.

- Ease of use
- Training and after sales services
- Cost to the patient
- Start up cost.

In evaluating an implant system, the clinician must inquire:
- Were animal experiments conducted before the implant system was marketed?
- Were progressive clinical trials undertaken?
- Are the results of at least 5 years long trials published in reputed journals?
- Have there been multicenter replication studies?

The clinician should realize that it is not valid to extrapolate results from one product to another merely on the basis of some superficial morphologic resemblance. The composition of the material, its purity, its surface characteristic and its preparation are of vital importance.

BONE BIOLOGY, IMPLANT HEALING AND THE IMPLANT TISSUE INTERPHASE

Surgical Wound Healing after Osteotomy and Implant Placement

Osteophylic Phase

When an implant is first placed into bone a blood clot forms around the implant. Titanium is a light weight non-noble metal that is corrosion resistant as the result of the formation of surface oxides. The biologic inertness of this oxide leads to the implants being so biocompatible. The body does not react to the oxides on titanium as a foreign object but recognize it immunologically as self.

It is important to inflict the least damage to the bone and soft tissues while drilling and placing implants. Sharp drills and proper saline coolants are necessary to keep the temperature in the bone below 47°C for one minute.[2,3] After the blood clot has formed, there is generalized inflammation due to the surgical insult. However while the inflammatory phase is still on, a more mature vascular network forms around the implant during the first 3 weeks. In addition ossification also begins during the first week by the migration of osteoblasts from the periosteum and endosteal osteoblast from the walls of the osteotomy. The trauma of placing the implant also results in necrosis of a thin layer (0.5 mm to 1 mm) of peri-implant bone. There is a critical period at around 2 weeks when bone resorption exceeds bone formation resulting in lower degree of primary stability than that achieved at the time of placement. The inflammatory or osteophylic phase lasts for one month and results in the formation of weak cell rich woven bone which chemically bonds to the oxides of the titanium implant. Following the formation of woven bone, the remodeling phase starts at the end of 4 weeks.

Remodeling Phase

Osteoclasts and osteoblasts interact in a coordinated way to replace the weak woven bone into a more load bearing lamellar bone. The remodeling phase lasts for about 3 months. It is influenced by micro-movement (not more than 100 µ) between the bone and implant, and good vascular supply.[4] Under electron microscope, it is shown that there is an intimate contact between the bone and the implant surface oxides due to certain bone matrix proteins which act as binders.

Primary Stability

Primary stability or the initial rigid fixation of the implant to the bone is of prime importance for secondary osseointegration. An implant which is mobile at the time of placement will never achieve secondary osseointegration. By mobile we mean which moves inside the osteotomy and is not in close contact to the bone. It is different from an implant which is in close contact to the bone but only turns when you torque it (spinner). A spinner implant which has a moderately rough surface, e.g. Dentsply Sirona Implants Plus surface and Noble Biocare Implants—Anodic oxidation surface, can get subsequently osseointegrated. Most implant systems today use screw threads to gain primary stability. The presence of screw threads also help by transferring compressive forces to the surrounding cortical and cancellous bone which is favorable and leads to increased bone density.

OSSEOINTEGRATION

Osseointegration is the replacement of initial bone fixation of the implant with mature load bearing lamellar bone. The surface roughness of the implant especially the grit blasted and thermally acid etched (Dentsply Sirona Implants—Plus surface) are of immense benefit for faster and stronger laying of load bearing bone due to their osteoconductive surface.[5] The rough surface also leads to increased surface area on implant which helps in obtaining greater bone to implant contact (BIC). An additional advantage of the thermal acid etching is that in addition to increasing the surface roughness of the grit-blasted surface, it also cleans and removes foreign matter from the implant surface.

REFERENCES

1. Branemark PI, Adell R, Breine U, et al. Intra-osseous anchorage of dental prostheses. I: Experimental studies. Scand J Plast Reconstr Surg. 1969;3:81-100.
2. Eriksson AR, Albrektsson T. Temperature threshold levels for heat induced bone tissue injury: a vital-microscopic study in the rabbit. J Prosthet Den. 1983;50:101-7.
3. Eriksson AR, Albrektsson T. The effect of heat on bone regeneration: an experimental study in rabbits using the bone growth chamber. J Oral Maxillofac Surg. 1984;42:705-11.
4. Szmukler-Moncler S, Piattelli A, Favero GA, Dubruille JH. Considerations preliminary to the application of early and immediate loading protocols in dental implantology. Clin Oral Implants Res. 2000;11:12-25.
5. Neugebauer J, Weinlander M, Lekovic V, et al. Mechanical stability of immediately loaded implants with various surfaces and designs: a pilot study in dogs. Int J Oral Maxillofac Implants. 2009;24(6):1083-92.

Chapter 2

Diagnosis and Treatment Planning

INTRODUCTION

The key to success of any dental treatment and more so with dental implant treatment is a well planned and preformed data-gathering process.

The treatment planning for implant supported prosthesis should begin with a clear idea of the end result which should fulfill the functional and aesthetic demands of the patient.

It is essential that all caries, endodontic lesions and periodontal diseases be treated before embarking on any implant treatment.

The minimal clinical examination should include the restorative status, periodontal screening, jaw relationship and occlusion.

The most convenient radiographic examination is the dental panoramic tomogram popularly known as OPG which stands for Ortho Pantomo Graphy (Fig. 2.1). This should be supplemented with intraoral radiographs for better image quality. Periapical radiographs should be considered for all heavily restored teeth, teeth with known or suspected endodontic problems and with periodontitis. Teeth with post-crowns should be carefully inspected for potential fracture of roots. Post-crown teeth as free-standing units may have a fair prognosis but should not be considered as abutment for fixed prosthodontics. Similarly, lateral incisors should not be considered as an abutment in a 4 unit fixed partial denture (Fig. 2.2).

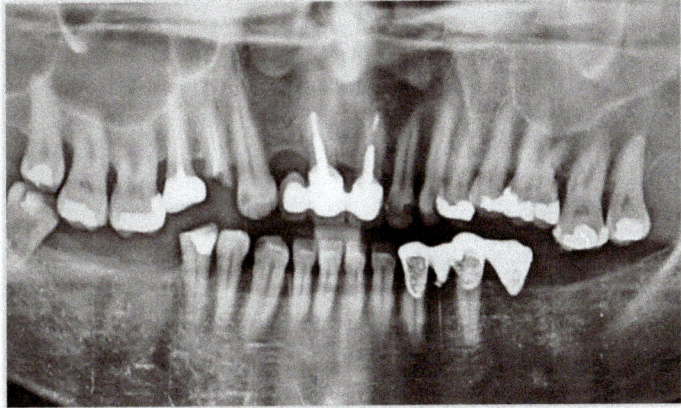

Fig. 2.1: OPG view of patient.

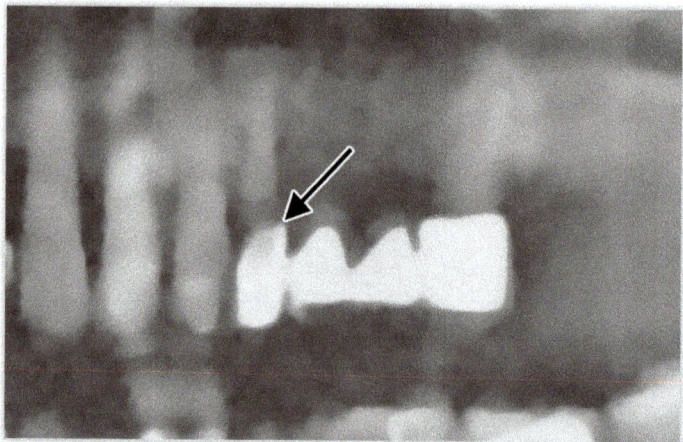

Fig. 2.2: Fracture of weak lateral incisor abutment.

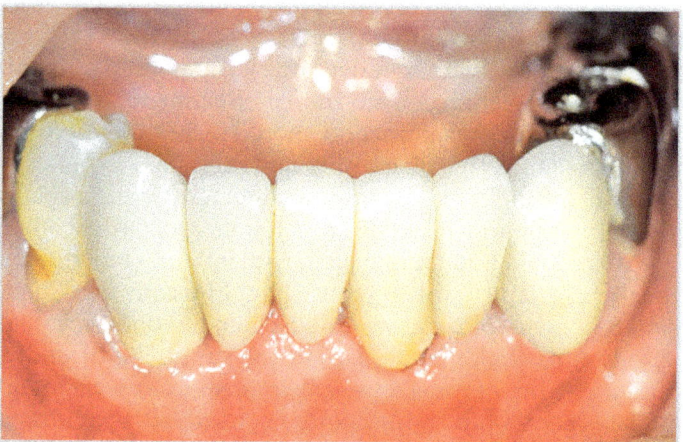

Fig. 2.3A: Implant supported fixed bridge.

The following type of implant retained restorations are possible:
- Fixed bridge (Figs. 2.3A and B)
- Over denture (Fig. 2.4)
- Single tooth restorations (Fig. 2.5).

IMPLANT-RETAINED FIXED BRIDGES

The prosthesis is similar in design to a conventional fixed bridge prosthesis constructed on natural teeth and can be screw retained or preferably cemented. Cantilevering fixed prosthesis more than one abutment anteriorly is not advised. However, in certain conditions, wherein we have multiple splinted implant abutments, it is possible to have 2 cantilevers in the non-functional anterior region (Figs. 2.6A and B).

Diagnosis and Treatment Planning

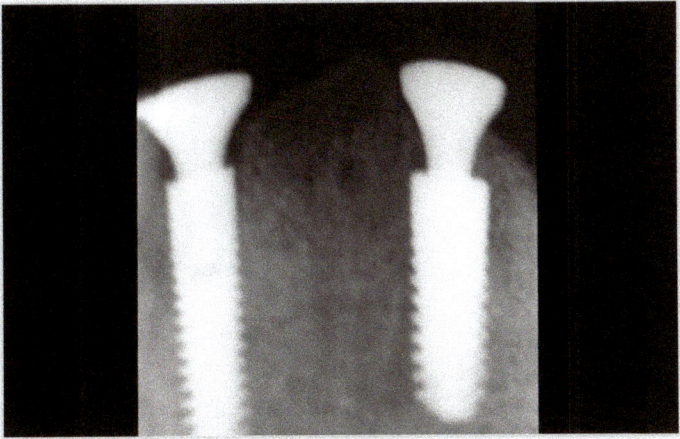

Fig. 2.3B: Radiographic view of implants before prosthetic rehabilitation.

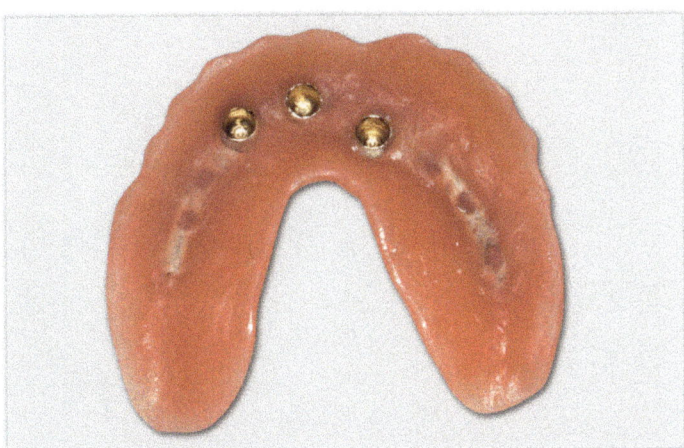

Fig. 2.4: Intaglio view of complete overdenture supported by 3 Syncone abutments.

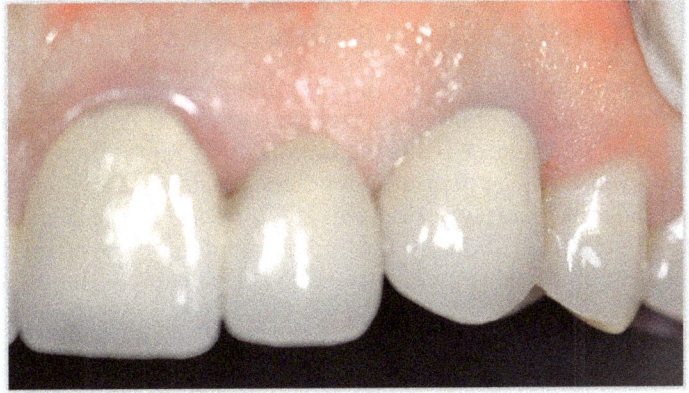

Fig. 2.5: Single implant supported crown on maxillary left canine.

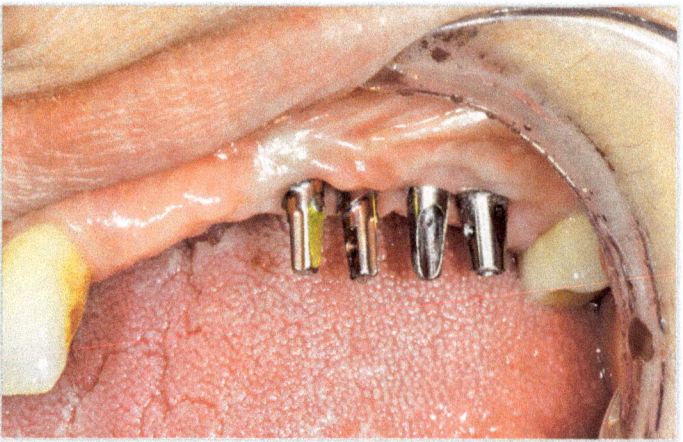

Fig. 2.6A: Four implants in the region of 24, 25, 26, 27.

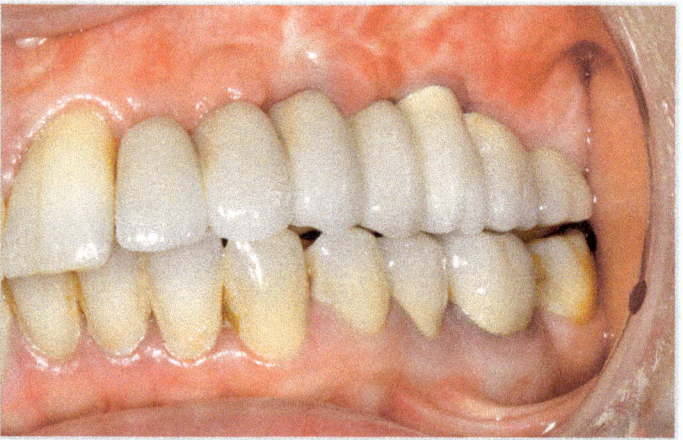

Fig. 2.6B: Implant supported fixed restorations with 2 anterior cantilevers.

IMPLANT-RETAINED OVERDENTURES

These are patient removable complete dentures usually with bar or ball attachment. In the mandible, it usually consists of two implants placed in the canine region with bar or ball attachments. Although it improves retention and stability of the lower denture, it is not the ideal solution, since, a mucosal-retained posterior causes continuous loss of bone in the posterior region. A better alternative is to have four implant abutments (Syncone abutments Dentsply Implants) with prefabricated Syncone caps in the denture (Figs. 2.7A and B).

Maxillary overdentures should also have minimum four implant abutments. However, in certain cases with improved implant abutment connections such as in the Ankylos system (Dentsply Implants), it is possible to work with only 3 implant abutments (Figs. 2.8A and B).

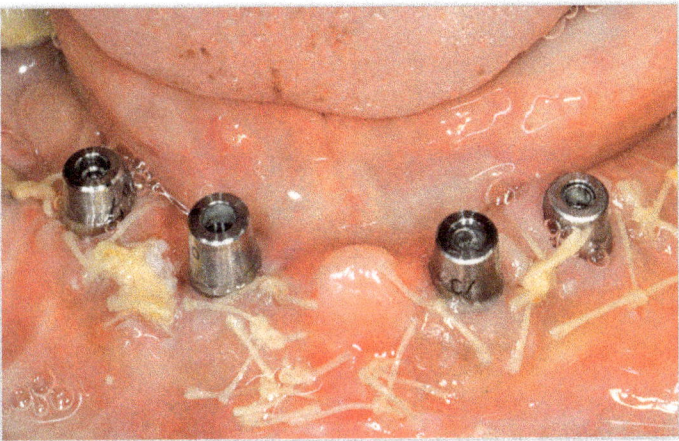

Fig. 2.7A: Ankylos implants with Syncone abutments on the day of surgery.

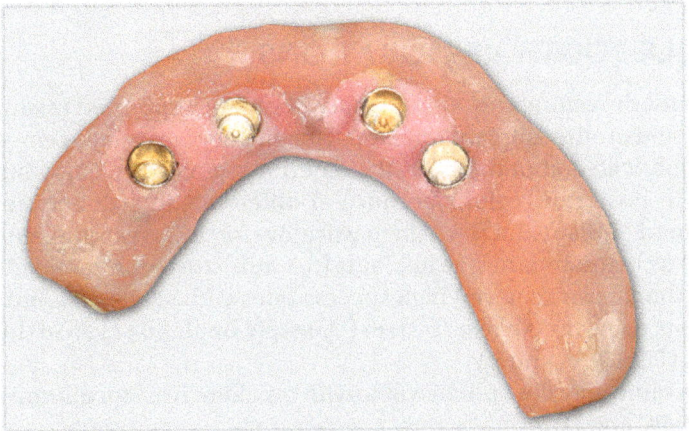

Fig. 2.7B: Four Syncone caps picked up in denture with self-cure acrylic on the day of surgery.

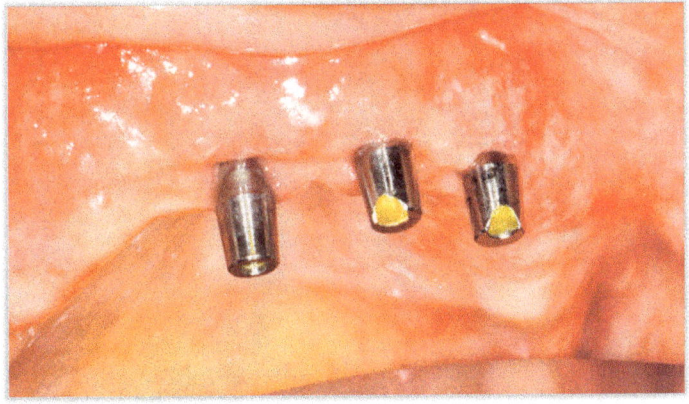

Fig. 2.8A: Three ankylos implants with 6° tapered Syncone abutments after a healing period of 3 months.

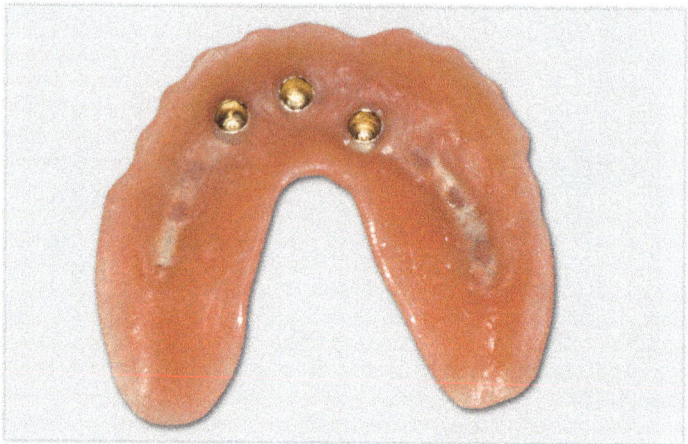

Fig. 2.8B: Syncone caps with cast metal frame work incorporated in complete maxillary denture.

SINGLE TOOTH RESTORATIONS

Single tooth restorations are individual implant supported restorations not connected to other implants or natural teeth. They are usually cement retained to prefabricated abutments. In the anterior region, they enjoy high success rates. In posterior regions because of difference in size between missing tooth, and implant and the high masticatory forces, larger implants (5 mm or 6 mm) or two standard size implants (3.5 mm) are recommended. However, the authors have achieved high success rates with single (4.5 mm diameter) implants using the Ankylos system (Dentsply Implants) even in the posterior region (Figs. 2.9A and B).

The same may not be achievable with butt joint implant abutment systems (Figs. 2.9C and D)

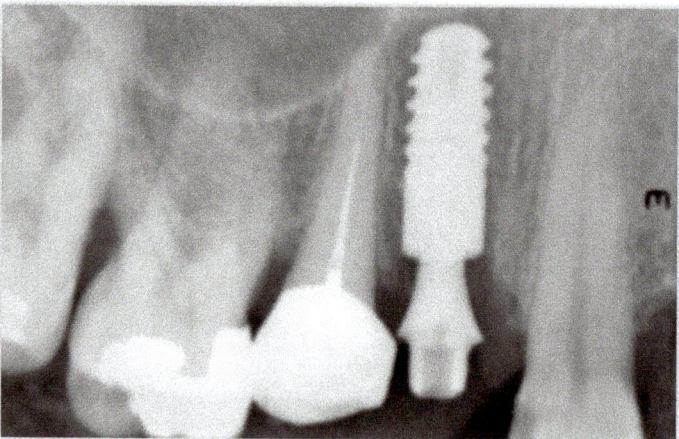

Fig. 2.9A: Ankylos implant with abutment on the day of surgery.

Diagnosis and Treatment Planning

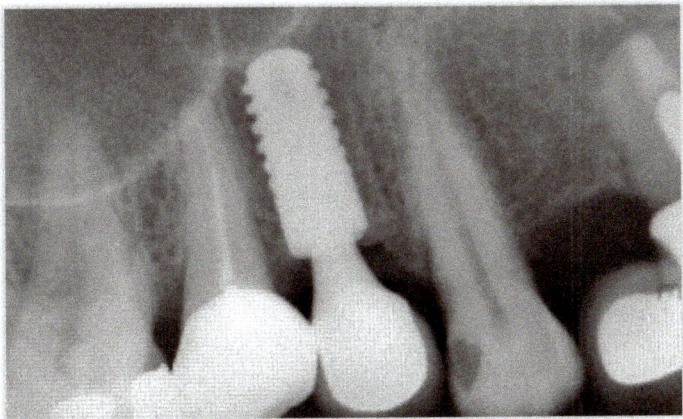

Fig. 2.9B: Ankylos implant after a loading period of 2 years. Note excellent crestal bone stability.

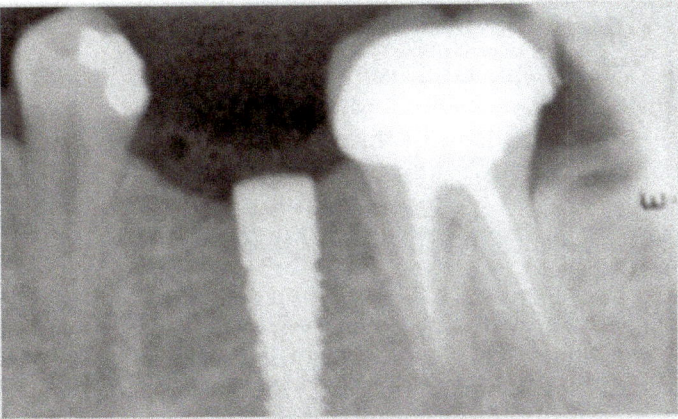

Fig. 2.9C: Implant placed on the day of surgery.

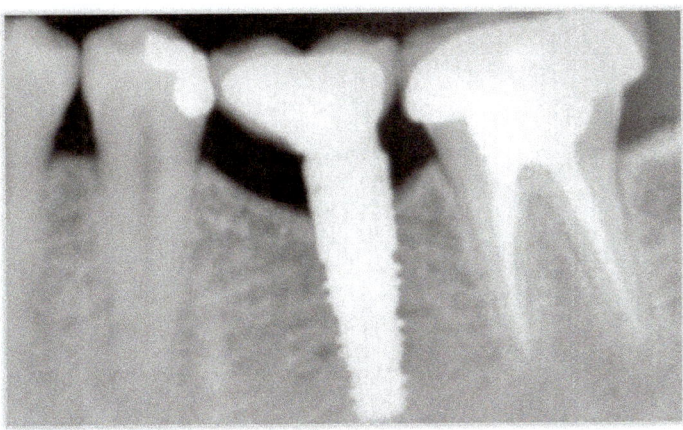

Fig. 2.9D: Same implant with butt joint implant abutment connection after 2 year. Note saucerization of the crestal bone.

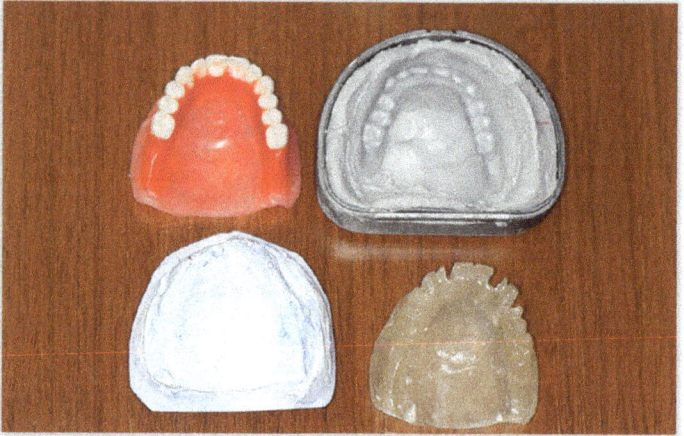

Fig. 2.10: Step in preparation of surgical stent.

PLANNING CONSIDERATIONS

Planning should commence keeping in mind the aesthetic and functional requirements of the patients. It should then proceed in more detail with intraoral examination, radiographic assessment, study cast, diagnostic wax-up and surgical stents (Fig. 2.10).

FUNCTIONAL CONSIDERATIONS

Inability to masticate food is a common complaint of patients who have lost their posterior teeth or who may be wearing removable dentures. The stability and retention of dentures can be improved by making them implant supported. If enough bone is present in the posterior region the patient can even opt for a fixed implant supported bridge instead of a removable denture (Figs. 2.11A and B).

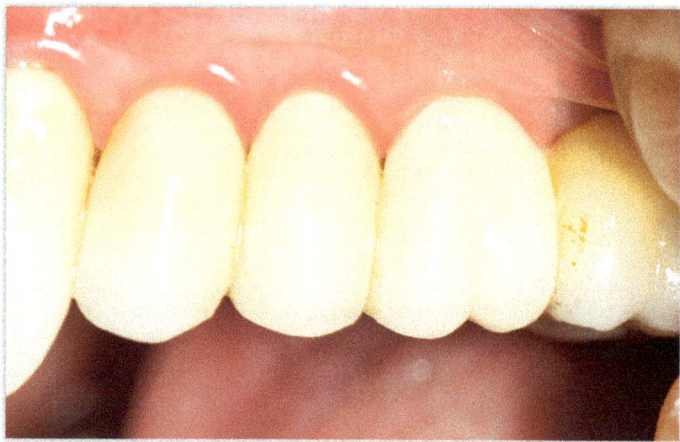

Fig. 2.11A: Fixed implant supported prosthesis.

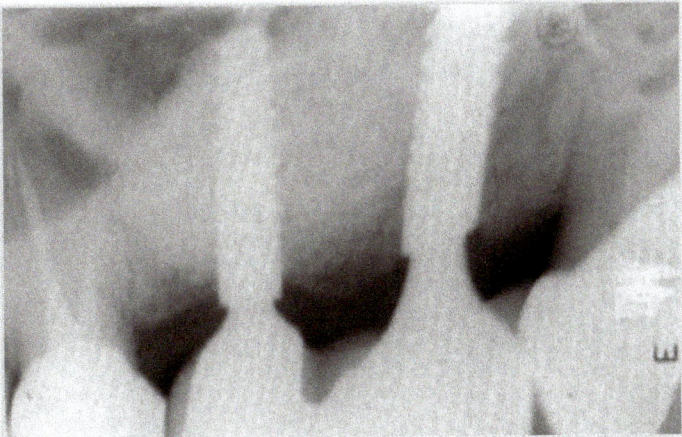

Fig. 2.11B: Radiographic view of the implant supported prosthesis done after lateral window sinus lift.

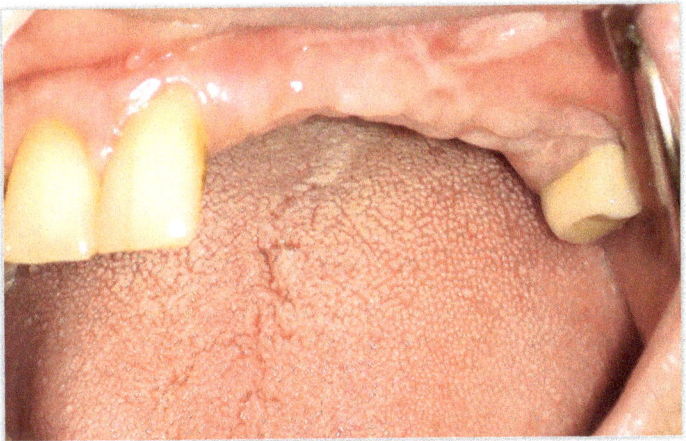

Fig. 2.12: Without provisional removable partial denture.

AESTHETIC CONSIDERATIONS

In some patients, aesthetic consideration plays a important role. It is important to note the amount of coverage of the anterior teeth and the gingiva by the lips of the patient at rest and also during smiling. Patients exhibiting a high smile line in which more teeth and gingiva are visible during smiling extra care should be taken. The patient should be examined with and without the current removable or fixed provisional denture to asses facial contour, lip support, teeth position and how much of the teeth are visible during function (Figs. 2.12 and 2.13).

On evaluation of the edentulous ridge, the height, width, contour and deficiencies can be visibly seen and manually palpated to assess their quality for implantation. The presence of deficiencies especially on the labial and

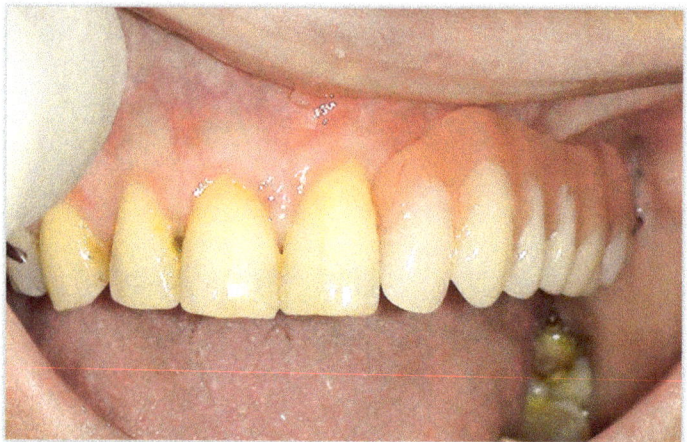

Fig. 2.13: With provisional removable partial denture.

buccal aspects of the ridge are readily apparent. However, the exact width of the bony ridges underneath the thick soft tissue, especially the palatal fibrous tissues cannot be accurately determined by just palpation. Ridge mapping using especially designed calibrated calipers (Fig. 2.14A) or by using graduated periodontal probes or endodontic files with stoppers are highly recommended in absence of computerized tomograms[1] (Fig. 2.14B).

STUDY CAST AND DIAGNOSTIC SET-UP

Articulated study casts help the clinician in making detailed measurements of many factors which are to be considered in the treatment plan (Fig. 2.15).

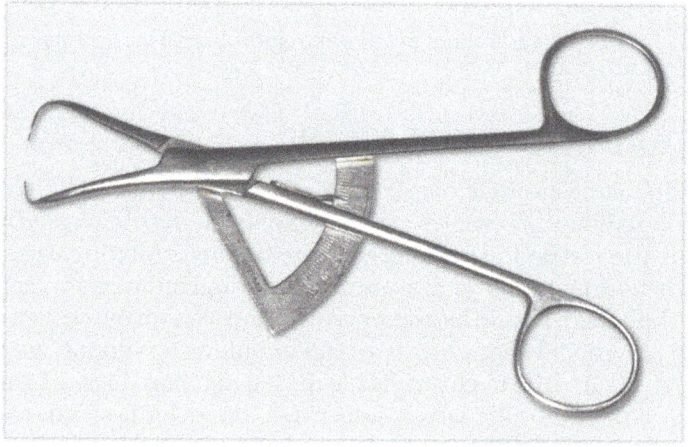

Fig. 2.14A: Especially designed calibrated caliper.

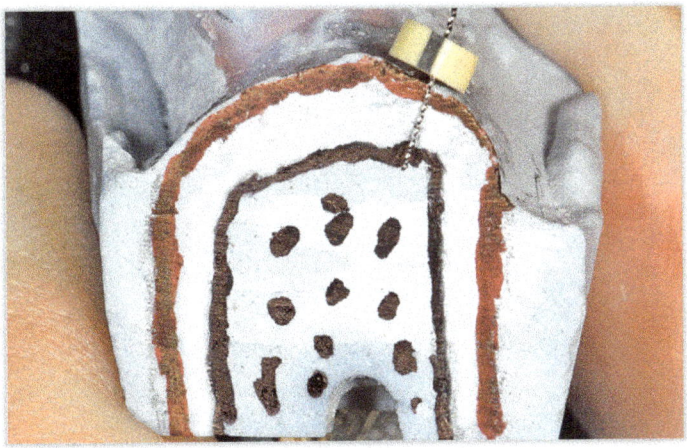

Fig. 2.14B: Ridge mapping done with the aid of endodontic file.

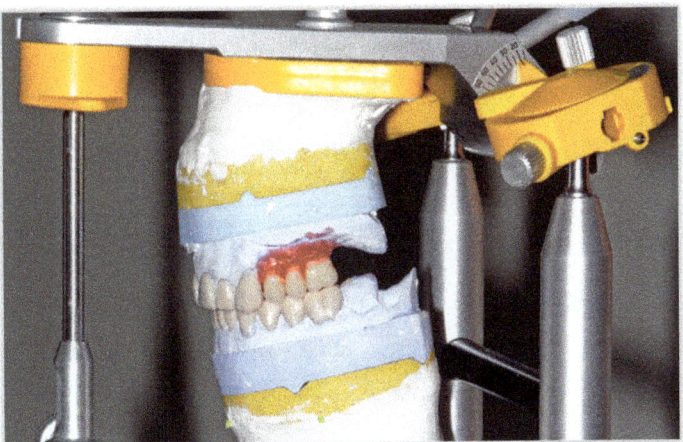

Fig. 2.15: Articulated study cast.

The teeth to be replaced can be positioned on the cast by wax build ups using denture teeth. The diagnostic set-up therefore helps in determining the number and position of the implants to be placed and also the future prosthodontic rehabilitation. It also helps in determining the occlusal relationship with the opposing dentition. Once the diagnostic step is ready, it can be used to prepare a blow-down surgical stent (Fig. 2.16). The blow-down stent could also have radiopaque markers in areas where implants need to be placed. The patient then wears the stent with the markers and gets an panoramic radiograph taken (Figs. 2.17A and B).

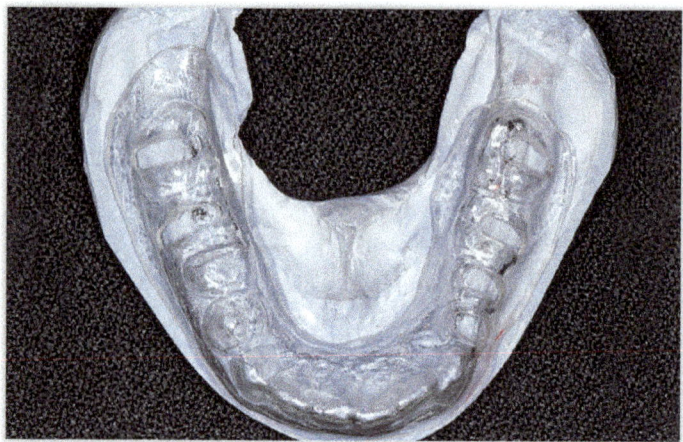

Fig. 2.16: Blown down surgical stent.

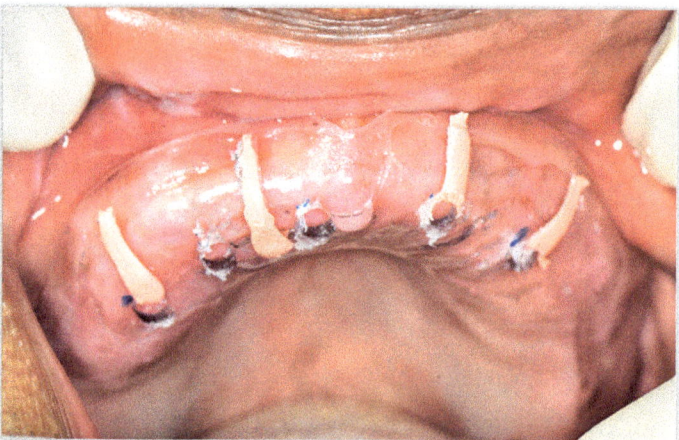

Fig. 2.17A: Stent with radiographic markers.

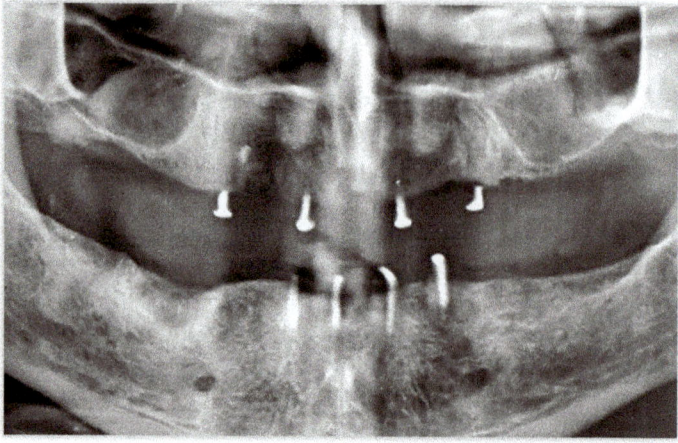

Fig. 2.17B: OPG showing radiographic markers.

IMPLANT SIZE, NUMBER AND SPACING

As a general guideline, one should replace each missing tooth by an implant. However in many situations, if this rule is followed implants would be placed too close to each other, which is not advisable. For all butt joint implant abutment connection implant systems, atleast 3 mm distance between two implants and 1.5 mm from adjacent natural teeth is required. This rule can be relaxed for conical taper connections such as the Ankylos system (Dentsply Implants) which allows implants to be placed closer to each other.[2]

The implant size namely diameter and length is determined from the radiographs, ridge mapping or still better cone beam computed tomography (CBCT). Implant size should be selected to ensure optimum stability. However, the largest diameter need not be selected. At least 1 mm of bone palatally, lingually and more importantly buccally should be kept to prevent resorption of thin plates of bone.[3]

ABSOLUTE MEDICAL CONTRAINDICATIONS

Implants should not be placed in patients with disease which compromise the ability of the tissue to heal. Patients on chemotherapy for treatment of cancer or antimetabolic therapy and for treatment of conditions such as arthritis should not be considered, as also severely impaired cardiovascular function.[4] Patients undergoing radiotherapy for cancer should also be avoided for implant treatment.

RELATIVE CONTRAINDICATIONS

Patients with cardiac and vascular disease, diabetes, osteoporosis have to be treated with caution and conventional precaution should be taken throughout surgical procedures, however, the above should not be considered as absolute contraindication. Heavy smokers are at great risk and all attempts should be made to stop or reduce smoking to ensure good healing.

PATIENTS ON BIPHOSPHONATE THERAPY

Biphosphonate therapy is usually prescribed for female patients who suffer from osteoporosis. There have been sporadic cases reported of osteonecrosis after placement of implants for a few of these patients. The reported cases have usually been associated with intravenous biphosphonate therapy. Therefore, it is recommended that patients who have been treated with intravenous biphosphonate therapy should be considered as absolute contraindications for implant surgery.

PSYCHIATRIC CONTRAINDICATIONS

Schizophrenic patients as also patients with severe paranoia should be excluded. Severe character disorders and neurotic syndromes are contraindications for treatment. Drug and alcohol abuse would impair patient compliance, and oral hygiene motivation which are needed for implant success.

REFERENCES

1. Wilson DJ. Ridge mapping for determination of alveolar riged width. Int J Oral Maxillifac Implant. 1989,4:41-3.
2. Vaitatic F, Belser U. Replacement of 4 missing upper incisons with standared or narrow neck implants: Analysis of different treatment options. Eur J Esthet. Dent. 2007:2:44-59.
3. Grunder U, Gracis S, Capelli M. Influence of the 3-D bone-to-implant relationship on esthetions. Int J Periodontics Restorative Dent. 2005:25:113-9.
4. Matsura H. systemic management of cardiovascular risk patients in dentistry. Anesth Pain Control Dent. 1993;2:49-61.

Chapter 3

Basic Implant Surgery

Although in this article the basic implant surgery is related to the Ankylos Implant System (Dentsply Sirona Implant) in partially edentulous subjects, the principles outlined will relate to all Implant systems. To achieve osseointegration a precise and low trauma surgical technique is essential. The diagnostic set up, surgical stent and relevant radiographs should be available. The surgeon should have a clear idea of the number, size and planned locations of the implants as explained in the previous article. Besides the planned implants an adequate stock of implants should be kept ready for any eventualities arising during surgery.

These are mandatory requisites because success in implant surgery will largely depend upon meticulous preoperative planning.

The surgeon should have adequate training in the procedure and should be able to handle any unforeseen circumstances.

SURGICAL PROTOCOL

The surgical protocol to be followed is:
- Good operating light
- Good high volume suction (Fig. 3.1A)

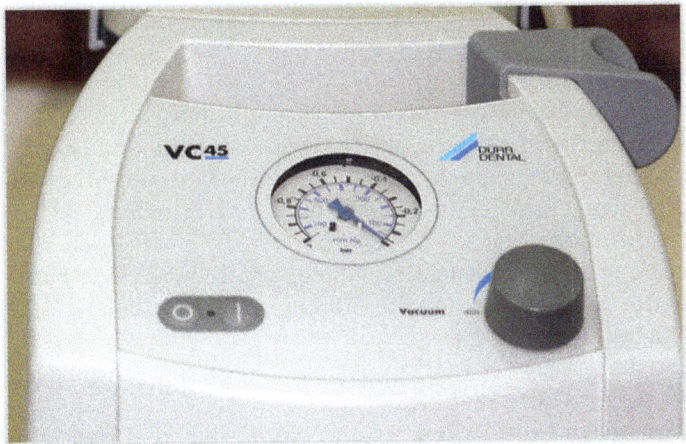

Fig. 3.1A: Surgical suction unit.

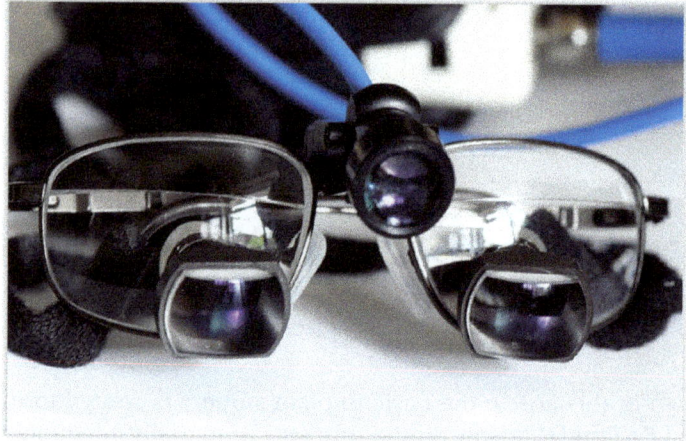

Fig. 3.1B: Magnifying loops with mounted LED light.

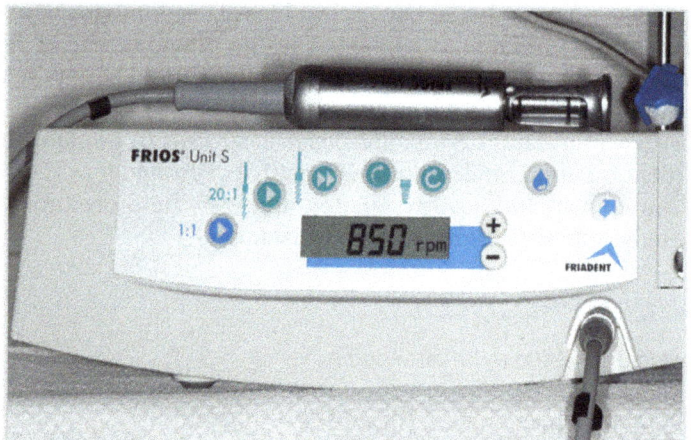

Fig. 3.1C: Surgical torque control motor.

- It is very important to work under Through-the-lens (TTL) magnification with an attached LED light, e.g. Designs for Vision, USA (Fig. 3.1B).
- A good dental chair which can be adjusted by foot control or by an assistant.
- A surgical unit with good control of torque, e.g. Frios Surgical Unit, Dentsply Sirona Implants (Fig. 3.1C).
- A properly designed irrigation system which can deliver chilled saline to keep the bone cool during the drilling, e.g. Frios Coolant Hoze, Dentsply Sirona Implants.
- Sterile drapes, gowns, masks, caps, suction tubing and gloves.
- Mayo surgical table (Fig. 3.1D)
- Preoperative mouthwash and perioral skin disinfection with 0.1% chlorhexidine, Periogard, Colgate, India (Fig. 3.1E).

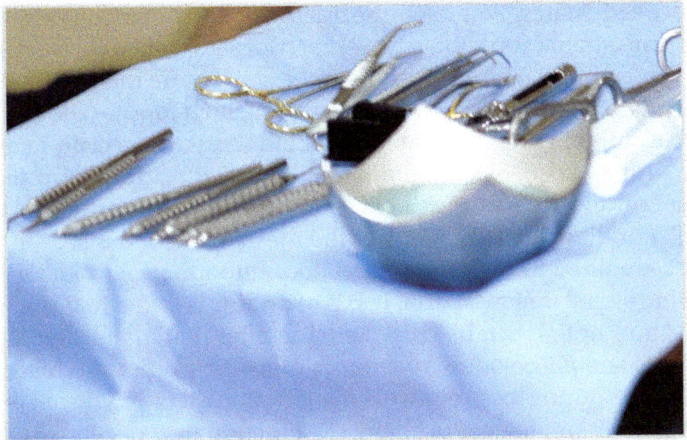

Fig. 3.1D: Mayo tray—surgical setup.

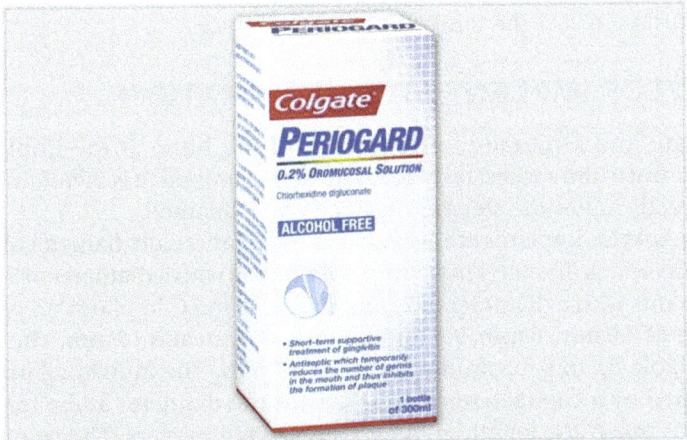

Fig. 3.1E: Chlorhexidine 0.12% (Periogard, Colgate, India).

- Antibiotic prophylaxis (Amoxycillin 500 mg plus clavulanic acid 125 mg (Tresmox CV Abbott). The authors prefer to supplement the above regime with an anaerobic chemotherapeutic agent, Metronidazole 400 mg (Pfizer, India). Patients allergic to the above should be prescribed Clindamycin 300 mg (Dalacin Pfizer). The antibiotics are taken orally 60 minutes before surgery.
- It is a good idea to give analgesic, e.g. diclofenac 100 mg plus paracetamol 325 mg along with serratiopeptidase 10 mg (Ebility, Abbott) prior to extensive surgery three times a day. The addition of serratiopeptidase helps in reducing soft tissue inflammation and swelling.
- In cases of lengthy surgeries with augmentation procedures the antibiotics may be continued in a dose of three times a day for 5-7 days.
- Most implant surgeries can be performed under local infiltration anesthesia with oral anxiolytic agents like clonazepam 0.5 mg (Abbott) taken 60 minutes before surgery. However, some patients will require intravenous conscious sedation with the assistance of a qualified anesthetist.

- Low speed drilling. Preferably the drilling speed should not exceed 850 rpm.
- The drills should continuously be kept cool with chilled sterile saline, so that the temperature in the bone does not exceed more than 47°C per minute.[1]
- The motor should be capable of delivering high torque (see Fig. 3.1C).
- An intermittent drilling technique should be used especially in dense bone.
- The drilling sequence should be incremental starting from the smallest twist drill and progressively enlarging the osteotomy to the final drill width.
- Whilst drilling tilt drill slightly in the mesial direction just as in nature the teeth are tilted in the mesial direction. Important not to alter the axis of drilling after 2 mm twist drill. If axis of drilling is found to be incorrect after the 2 mm drill, it can be corrected, but after that, no further alteration of the axis should be done or chances of losing primary stability will arise. Therefore, during the process of enlarging the osteotomy do not put pressure on the drills or chances of changing direction may result. Take the help of associates or nurses to help you in determining the correct axis.
- Change drills once you find they have lost their sharpness. Do not use same drills after 20 drillings. Dull drills require greater pressure on them which in turn increases the temperature in the bone.

ANKYLOS IMPLANT SITE PREPARATION

Accurate and atraumatic preparation of the bone at the implant site is paramount to the successful placement of the implant. It is therefore important to correctly follow the steps as outlined and explained.

The Ankylos implants are available as A implants with diameter of 3.5 mm, B implants with a diameter of 4.5 mm, C implants with a diameter of 5.5 mm and D implants with a diameter of 7 mm. The A, B and C implants are available in lengths of 6.6 mm, 8 mm, 9.5 mm, 11 mm, 14 mm and 17 mm. The D implant is available up to a maximum length of 14 mm. The individual implants are identified by a capital letter that indicates the diameter and a number. The number shows the length of the implant in millimeters. The color coding of the implant package identifies the implant diameter. The drills, reamers and taps are also color coded.

The patented thread design of the Ankylos implant is designed to match the structure density of the bone.
- The cervical geometry of the thread (shallow threads) reduces load transfer to the cortical crestal bone (Fig. 3.2).
- Continuously increasing depths of the thread (towards the apical) transfers load to the cancellous bone (Fig. 3.2).
- The square shape of the Ankylos threads load the bone interphase in compression when an axial load is delivered. Bone is strongest when loaded in compression. The square thread also results in less stress on occlusal loading in all bone densities (Fig. 3.3).

Studies have shown that a rough microtextured implant surface gives rise to higher bone to implant contact than machined implants. However early designs using an additive process like 'Plasma Spraying' or Hydroxyl Apatite (HA) Coating although improved bone to implant contacts, had disadvantages

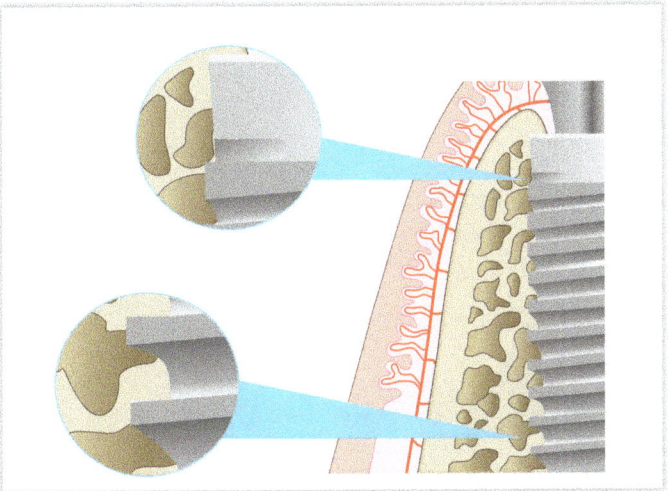

Fig. 3.2: Cervical threads are shallow to reduce stress in crestal bone. Apical threads are deeper to transfer compression in trabecular bone.

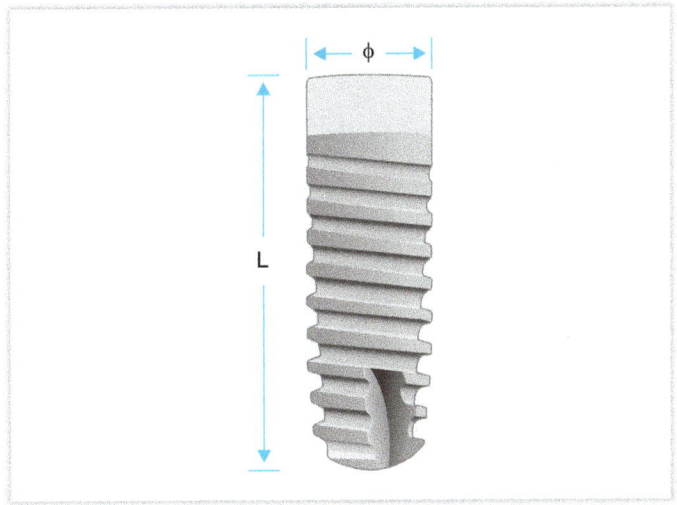

Fig. 3.3: Outer surface of threads are square, thus loading the bone in compression.

such as flaking and cracking of the coatings on insertion. Also such coatings increased plaque adhesion and were more prone to peri-implantitis. A recently introduced technology of using sand blasting and computer controlled high temperature acid etching (Dentsply Implants Plus) results in a microstructure which has the following advantages:
- It has improved wetting properties which activates primary osteoblast deposition and subsequent optimum osseointegration in the shortest possible time (Fig. 3.4).

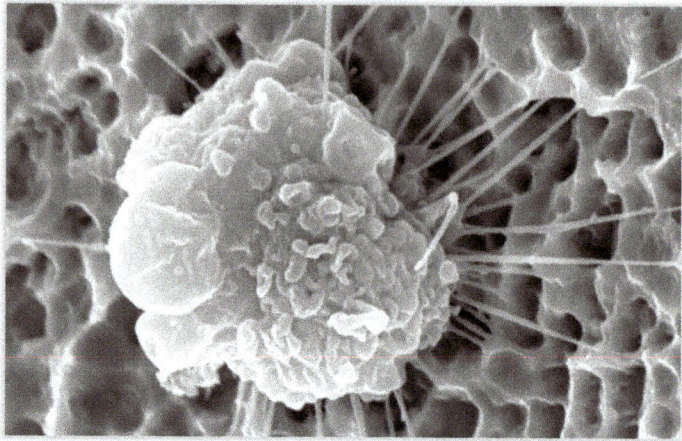

Fig. 3.4: Osteoblast deposition and spreading on the microtextured surface.

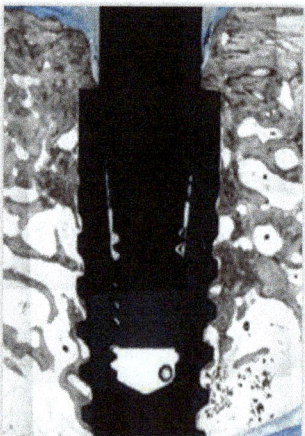

Fig. 3.5: Histomorphometric view showing bone deposition over the shoulder of the Ankylos Implant.

- The other unique feature of the Ankylos Implants is the lack of smooth collar on the implant. A special surface treatment on the cervical margin and the end face means that bone can form even on the horizontal shoulder of the implant, thus providing additional support for the soft tissues. (Fig. 3.5)

PLACEMENT OF AN ANKYLOS IMPLANT IN STANDARD POSTERIOR SITES: STEP-BY-STEP PROCEDURES

Reflection of Mucoperiosteal Flaps

- The surgery begins with a mid-crestal incision made with a no. 15 surgical blade. The rationale for this type of incision is to maintain equal amount of keratinized tissue on the buccal and lingual sides. Incisions wherever possible should be placed in attached gingiva (Fig. 3.6).

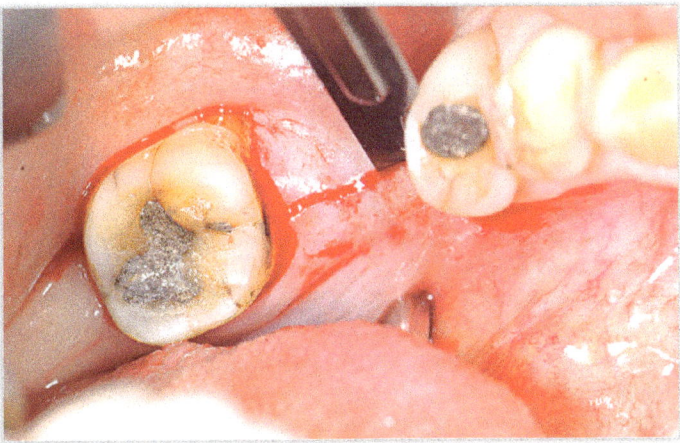

Fig. 3.6: Midcrestal incision with no.15 surgical blade.

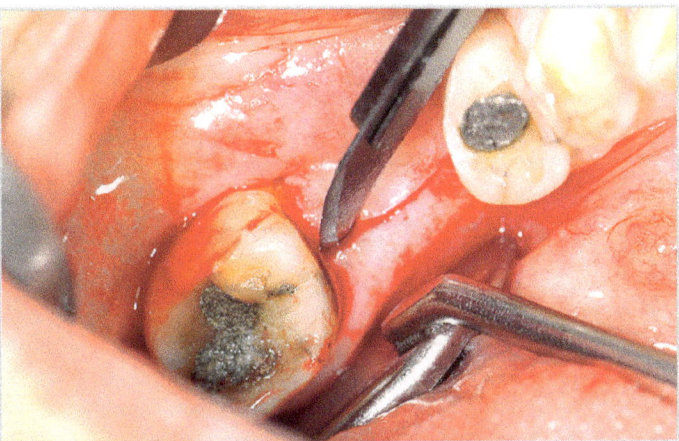

Fig. 3.7: 12B blade in use to extend incision up to adjacent teeth.

- A No. 12B blade which has cutting surfaces on both sides should be used to extend the incisions up to the tooth to prevent tearing of the flap during elevation (Fig. 3.7).
- Next extend your incision into the sulcus and the papillae with the no. 15C or 12B blade.

Always first use the papilla elevator and work into the marginal tissues to mobilize the flap. Follow it up with small sharp elevators to further mobilize the flap (Figs. 3.8A and B).

- Preferably first mobilize the lingual or palatal flap (Fig. 3.9) and then come to the buccal side, since the lingual or palatal is more easy to mobilize than the buccal (Fig. 3.10).
- It is better to start reflecting from anterior to posterior aspect.
- Avoid vertical incisions wherever possible since they take longer to heal and are uncomfortable and painful for the patients.

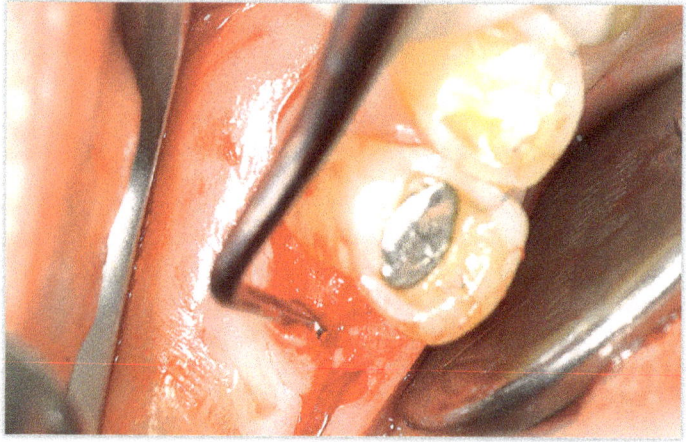

Fig. 3.8A: Papilla elevator reflecting marginal tissues.

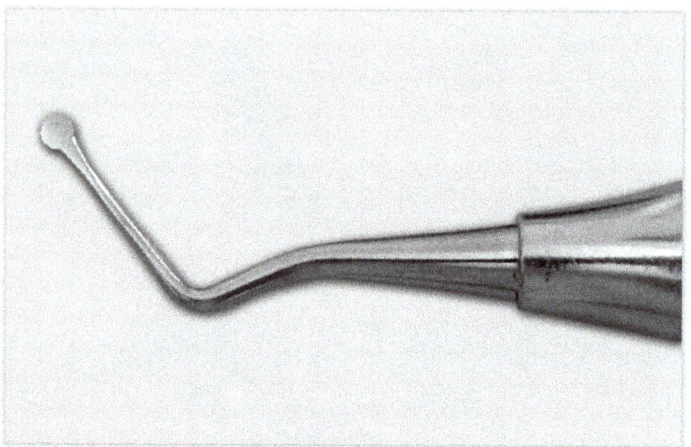

Fig. 3.8B: Discoid-shaped semi-sharp papilla elevator.

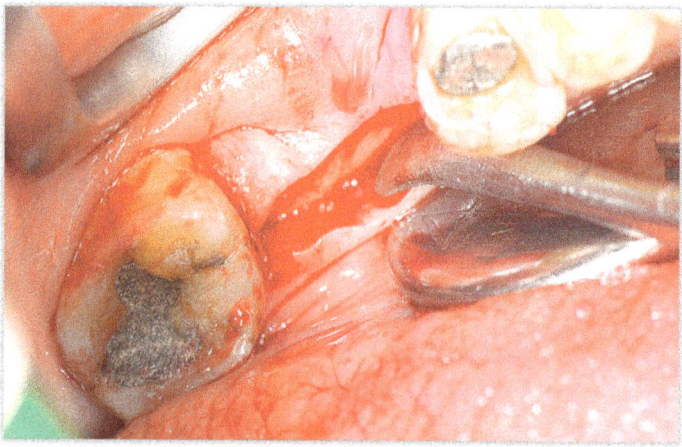

Fig. 3.9: Mobilization of lingual flap.

Basic Implant Surgery

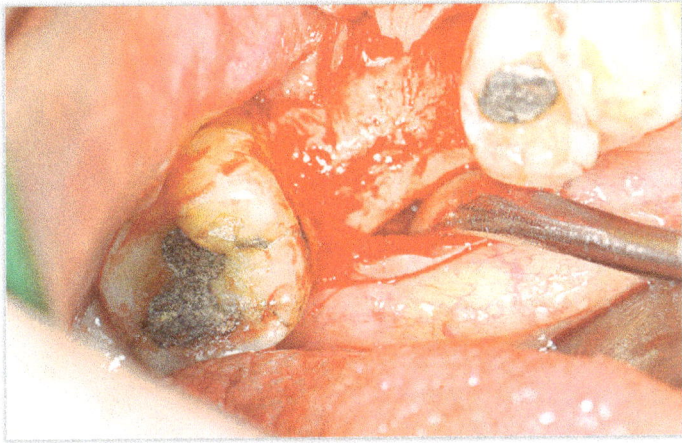

Fig. 3.10: Complete flap reflection.

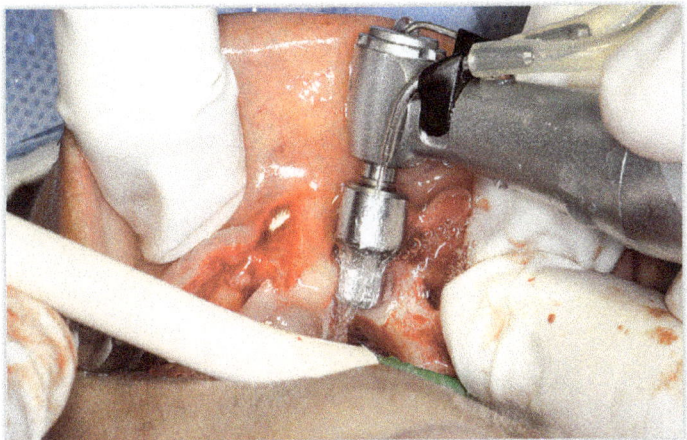

Fig. 3.11: Bone contouring bur to remove irregularities and level the ridge.

Leveling and Smoothening of the Crestal Ridge

Use a bone contouring bur (Salvin Dental Laxmi Associates, Chennai, Tamil Nadu, India) or a large round bur to remove irregularities and level the ridge. This step also helps in removing tissue remnants present on the bone (Fig. 3.11). A spacer tab is used to determine the distance of the anterior implant from the distal surface of the natural tooth (Fig. 3.12). The spacer tab does not replace the surgical stent but is an adjunct.

Osteotomy Preparation

The location of the implant on the crest of the ridge is marked with a small round bur or with a lance drill (MIS Implant) with the help of the surgical guide (Fig. 3.13). Use drills which allow internal as well as external cooling.

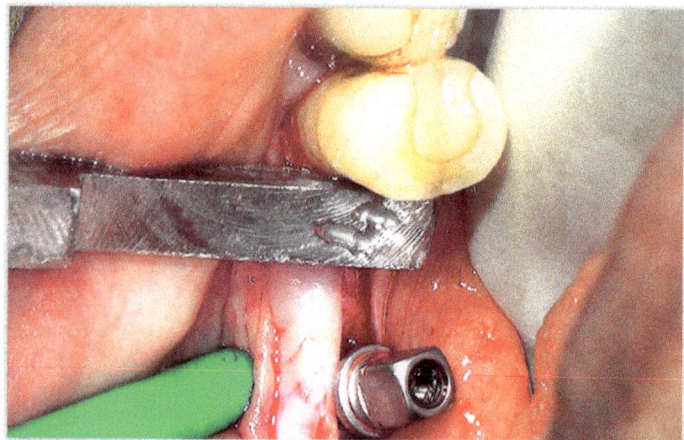

Fig. 3.12: Spacer tab in place.

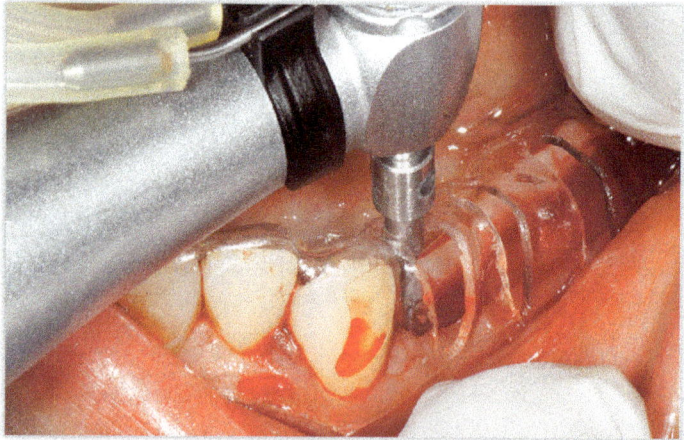

Fig. 3.13: Initial osteotomy with surgical guide and Lindemann drill.

All drills of the Ankylos system except the conical reamer and the tap are designed for internal and external cooling. However, bone debris may block the opening of the internal cooling, therefore one should check the drills at intervals outside the patients mouth to ensure that the coolant is still flowing. After each drilling, bone debris clinging to the drills should be wiped away with surgical gauge lightly moistened with 0.12% chlorhexidine (Periogard, Colgate India).

    The first 2.0 twist drill (pilot drill) is positioned and the site is prepared to a depth of 8 mm. The angulation of the implant axis is repeatedly checked with the help of direction indicators also known as Paralleling Guide Pins (Fig. 3.14) throughout the drilling process in relation to the surgical stent and the opposing dentition. The angulations should be checked from different

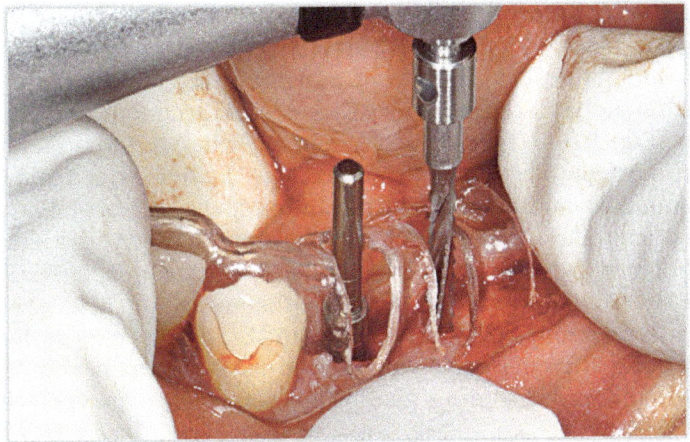

Fig. 3.14: Paralleling guide pins in anterior osteotomy and drill in posterior.

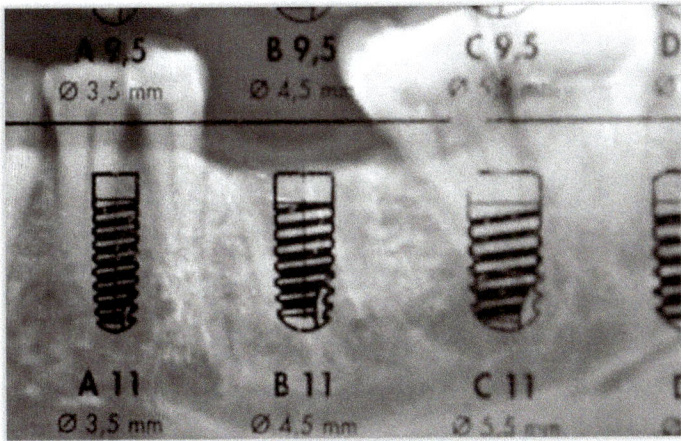

Fig. 3.15: Ankylos implant template placed on the OPG for selection of appropriate implant dimensions.

viewpoints buccal and occlusal as it is very easy to make a mistake if it is checked from one single aspect.

The implant lengths may be selected by (CBCT) or by placing the transparent radiographic template of the Ankylos system on the OPG (magnification 1:25) (Fig. 3.15). If desired and if anatomic structures permit, the X-ray analysis may consider a slightly (0.5 mm to 1 mm) subcrestal placement.

After the axis is confirmed, the 2 mm twist drill should be used to the final determined depth of the implant. The next drill according to the Ankylos system is the 3.5 mm Tri-spade drill which is taken to full length. However, the authors prefer an intermediate drill and therefore use the 2.75 mm Tri-spade drill from (Salvin Dental, Laxmi Associates, Chennai). The use of 2.75 mm drill before the 3.5 mm drill allows easy placement of the 3.5 mm drill, especially in dense bone.

The 3.5 mm Tri-spade drill is the final drill for the 3.5 mm implant, unless you plan to place a 4.5 mm or 5.5 mm implant and then you have to enlarge incrementally the osteotomy. However an important step of the Ankylos system is the coronal shaping of the drilled site, which is accomplished by the conical reamer (Fig. 3.16). The conical reamer according to the preference of the authors is usually placed with a Contra Angle Handpiece for A and B implants and manually for C implants. The maximum speed should be 15 rpm and the maximum torque should be 50 Ncm. The reamer is used with a light pressure. The noncutting tip ensures that the drilled hole is not deepened. The reamer is removed from the cavity while still rotating.

Manual operation of the reamer for C and D implants require the reamer to be attached to a ratchet insert which is then inserted into a ratchet. The pins on the open-end wrench assist in guiding the instrument to prevent it from tilting (Fig. 3.17).

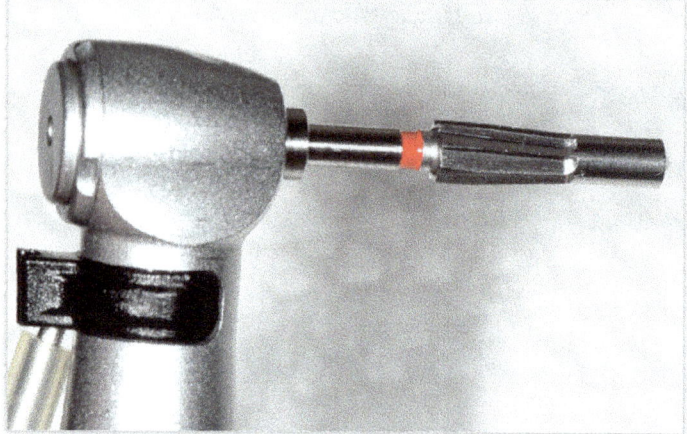

Fig. 3.16: Coronal shaping of the osteotomy with the conical reamer.

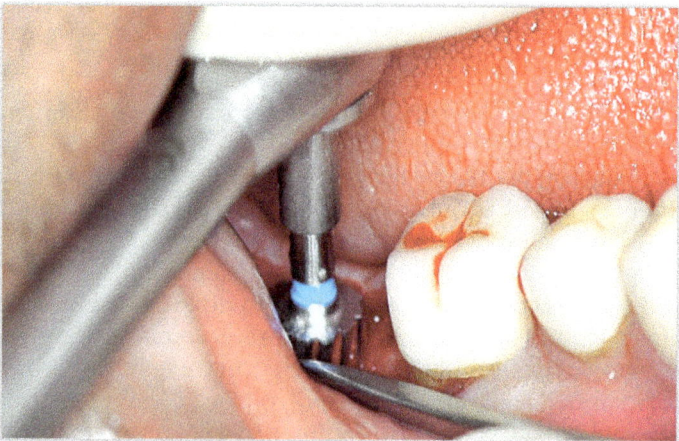

Fig. 3.17: Manual use of conical reamer for C implant with the wrench.

Salient Features of the Conical Reamer

The conical reamer allows you to gauge if you have drilled to the full depth. The margin of the reamer should be flushed with the bone crest or if subcrestal placement is planned, the margin should be slightly below the bone surface. (Fig. 3.18). If this is not the case, the implant site should be deepened to the required depth with the last used Tri-spade drill. The conical reamer is also an indispensable tool for:

a. Gauging whether your implant will have primary stability.
b. In some cases, it can be used as final preparation tool like an osteotome with the help of a especially designed instrument by Professor GH Nentwig. In certain conditions, the conical reamer works better than the smooth osteotome in preparing the surgical site to receive the implant (Fig. 3.19).

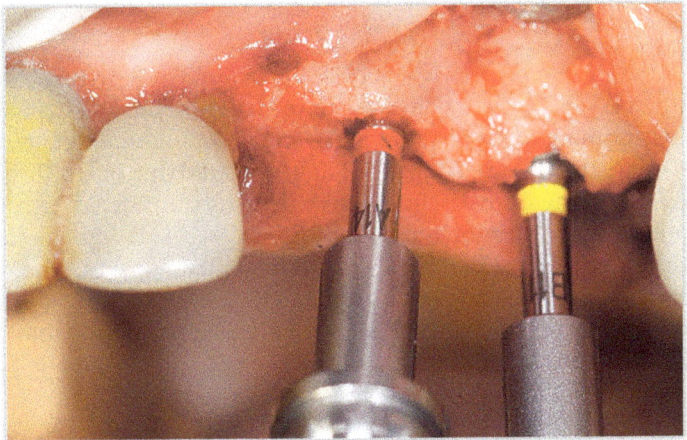

Fig. 3.18: Conical reamer flushed with the bone crest.

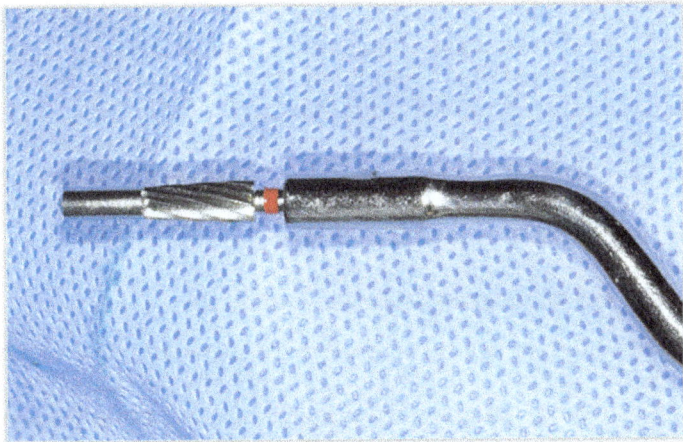

Fig. 3.19: Especially designed instrument by Professor GH Nentwig.

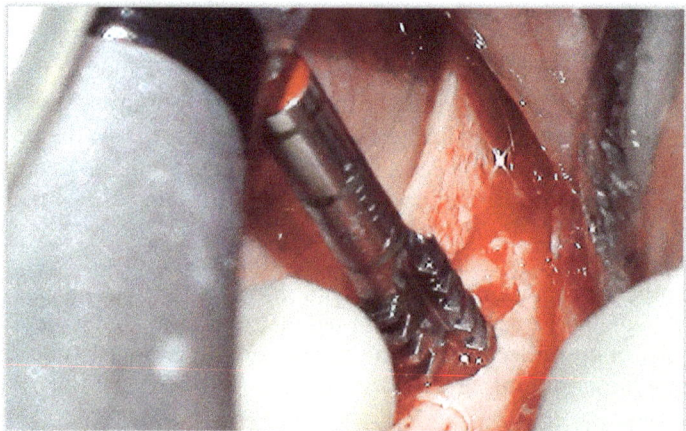

Fig. 3.20: Motorized use of the bone tap with a handpiece.

Tapping the Thread

Since the Ankylos Implants have a square-shaped thread design, the implant is not self-tapping except in very soft bone. It is therefore recommended to use the tap to the required depth but never beyond that or the threads will be stripped and this will adversely affect the primary stability. As with the reamer, the tap can be used motorized with a Contra Angle Handpiece (for A and B implants only) (Fig. 3.20) or with a manual ratchet.

As mentioned earlier, do not use the tap for D4 bone (very poor density) as you may adversely affect the primary stability. If used motorized, the reamer and tap should be used at a maximum speed of 15 rpm and at a maximum torque of 50 Ncm.

Ankylos Implant Placement

A and B implants can be placed by hand or motorized with the help of a Contra Angle Handpiece. It is important to note that to prevent heat necrosis, the rotation speed of the implant should not exceed 15 rpm.

It is recommended that A and B implants be placed by machine using a surgical unit with a torque measuring function (Frios Unit S/L, Dentsply Sirona Implants, Germany). Accurate torque measurement is essential for immediate function of implants. The maximum speed is 15 rpm and the maximum torque is 50 Ncm. If the implant becomes difficult to screw before it reaches its final position, unscrew it, rinse and tap the site.

Submerged or Transgingival Healing

The Ankylos implant can be kept submerged covered by a cover screw for undisturbed healing for a period of 2–3 months before second stage uncovering. However, if adequate primary stability is achieved (35 Ncm and above), it would be advantageous to cover the implant with a sulcus former of an appropriate height depending on the thickness of the gingiva (Fig. 3.21). With transgingival healing, a second surgical procedure is avoided, at the same time, you take

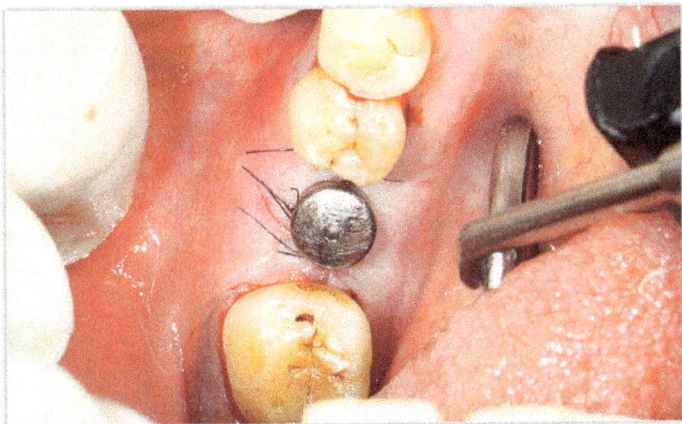

Fig. 3.21: Transgingival healing with the aid of sulcus former.

maximum advantage of the regenerative potential of the soft tissues to create an excellent emergence profile.

Surgical Procedure to Prepare Osteotomy in Compromised Bone

Poor quality bone (D3 and D4 Misch's classification)[2] is characterized by bone trabecular with little or no crestal cortical plate. In such situations, it is important to use only the pilot drill 2 mm or Lindemann drill and then enlarge the osteotomy by condensing the bone trabeculae with the sequential use of condensing osteotomes (Dentsply Sirona Implants, Germany) (Fig. 3.22). The idea being, you do not remove bone by drilling but rather condense it and improve the quality so that you can obtain primary stability of your implant.

It is also important in very poor quality bone to enlarge the osteotomy to one millimeter smaller than the diameter of the implant to be inserted. Although the Ankylos implant is not self-tapping, in poor quality of bone it will be able to self-tap its way to the final determined depth. The authors prefer to place the implant motorized with Contra Angle Handpiece at a speed of 15 rpm and maximum torque of 50 Ncm (Fig. 3.23). If the implant gets stuck and refuses to go further to the determined depth, unscrew it and enlarge the osteotomy with a larger osteotome or still better use the conical reamer with the Nentwig holder from Ustomed, Germany as an osteotome (Figs. 3.24A and B). It is important to avoid tapping the bone in poor quality for fear of losing primary stability. This type of bone is usually found in the posterior maxilla and sometimes also in posterior mandible.

Second Stage Surgery for Uncovering of Submerged Implants

Since the Ankylos implant has a conical morse taper implant abutment connection it requires minimum exposure of the soft tissues as this is mainly to gain access to the internal area of the morse taper.

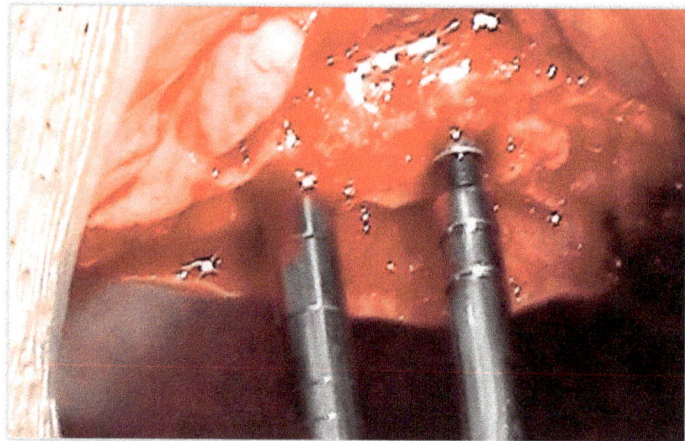

Fig. 3.22: Use of Osteotome to condense and enlarge the osteotomy

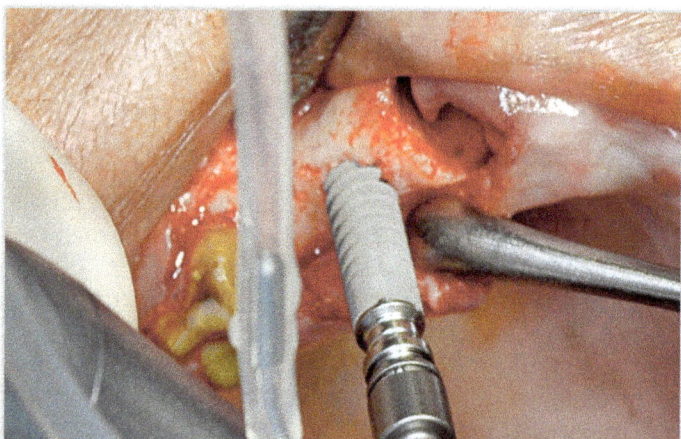

Fig. 3.23: Motorized insertion of Implant.

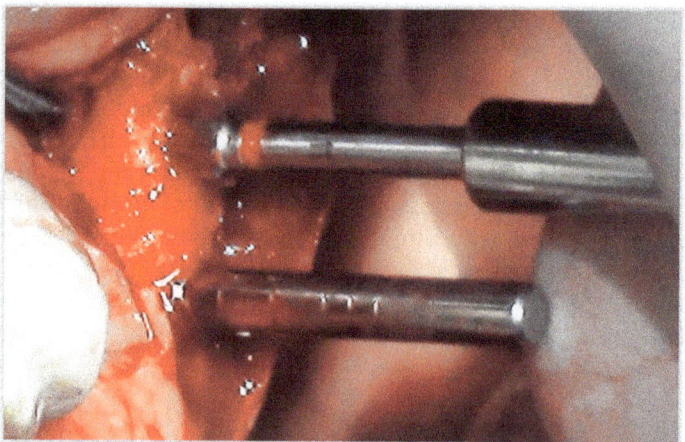

Fig. 3.24A: Use of conical reamer with Professor Nentwig's instrument.

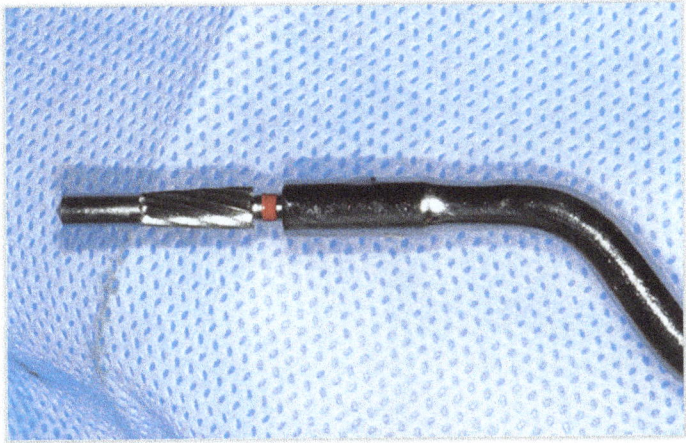

Fig. 3.24B: Especially designed instrument by Professor GH Nentwig.

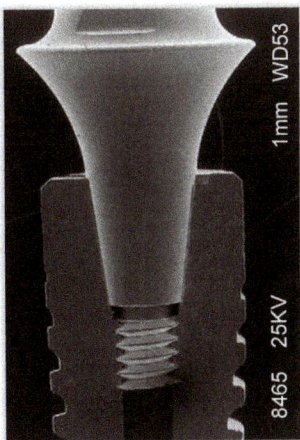

Fig. 3.25: Abutment fitting within the Implant.

The abutment does not have to be on top of the implant shoulder but fits within it (Fig. 3.25). The butt joint implant abutment connection requires the greatest amount of exposure and also great attention must be taken not to damage the implant shoulder especially so with external hex butt joints. The incision is usually mid crestal in the mandible and slightly to the palatal in the maxilla. Using small papilla elevators and small periosteal elevators the implant is exposed only as much as is required to place your unscrew instrument to remove the cover screw. The appropriate gingival height of sulcus former is then placed with the help of the 1 mm hex screw driver. In many instances, there is no need for sutures (Figs. 3.26A to D).

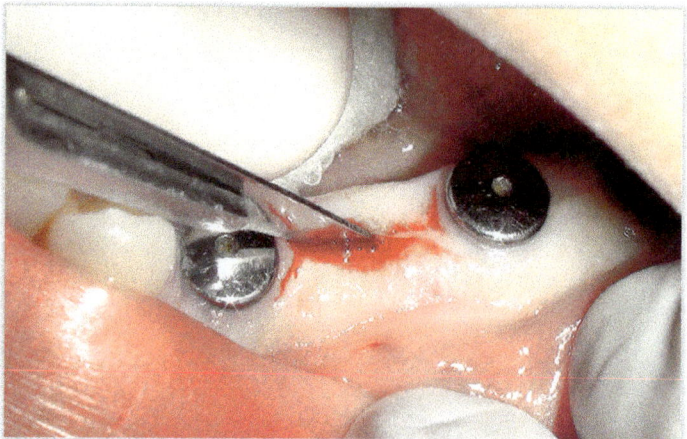

Fig. 3.26A: Initial incision for uncovering of implant.

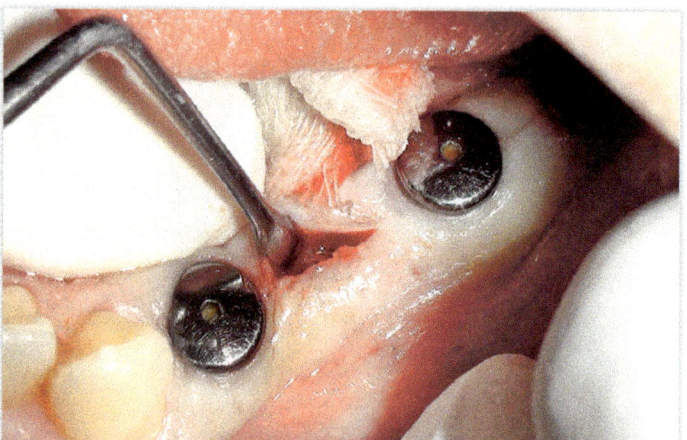

Fig. 3.26B: Small curette used to expose the cover screw of the implant.

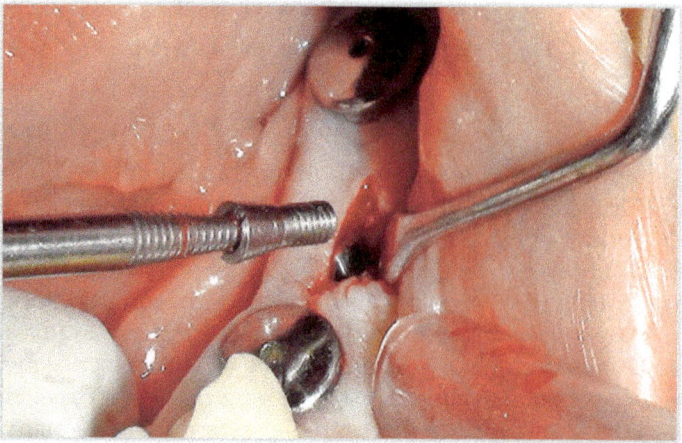

Fig. 3.26C: Unscrewing the cover screw from the implant.

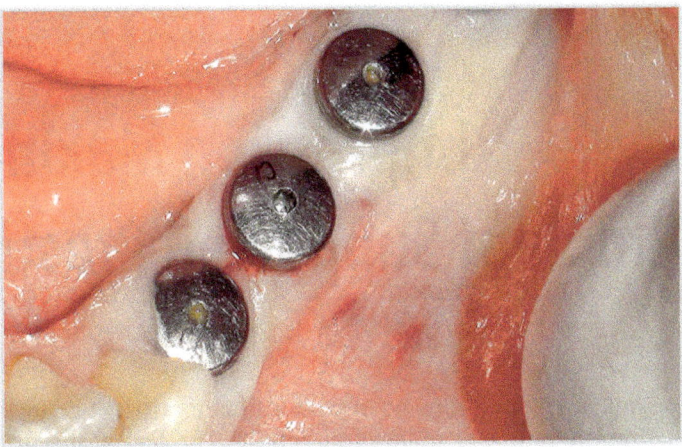

Fig. 3.26D: Sulcus former placed without need for suturing.

REFERENCES

1. Eriksson R, Albrektsson T. Temperature threshold levels for heat induced bone tissue injury: a vital-microscopic study in the rabbit. J Prosthet Den. 1983;50:101-7.
2. Misch CE. Density of Bone: Effects on surgical approach and healing, In: Misch CE. Contemporary Implant Dentistry. 2008:645-67.

Chapter 4

Impression Making for Implant Supported Prosthesis

Since the Ankylos system allows connecting implants to natural teeth (because of its strong implant abutment connection), the technique for recording impressions for prepared teeth as well as implants will be described.

The marginal fit of a restoration determines besides aesthetics, its clinical longevity in the mouth. Taking an accurate impression is an essential step in a well-fitting restoration. Several factors influence the recording of a prepared tooth or abutment:

GINGIVAL HEALTH

It is much easier to record an impression, if the gingiva is healthy. It is impossible to obtain a clear sharp impression, if there is a sea of blood and/or saliva. It is therefore, imperative to do a thorough subgingival scaling and curettage and wait for several days before taking an impression.

Proper Impression Tray

It is important to select a rigid impression tray, which locks the impression material (RIM-LOCK, Dentsply, India) or a perforated metal tray (Associated Dental, Mumbai). Be sure that no part of the tray touches the teeth. Use a tray adhesive.

Accurate Impression Material

Today, there are many excellent impression materials at our disposal. However, the top rated by 'Reality' is a hydrophilic, quadrafunctional modified vinyl polysiloxane, (Aquasil Ultra, Dentsply, India). Aquasil contains four reactive vinyl groups, which results in increased crosslinking of the polymer web than that obtained with conventional vinyl siloxanes. The tear strength is consequently improved. In addition, the proprietary surfactant results in significantly improved recording even in a wet environment and also results in superior cast reproduction. The improved wetting ability of the material is of great importance in recording surface details in the critical gingival sulcus area.

When a dentist has to impress 8–10 teeth, you need an impression material that has prolonged low characteristics during work time, Aquasil achieves that goal exceptionally well by its prolonged low characteristics during working time.[1]

Working Time

It is extremely important to work fast because once polymerization of the impression material starts, one should not record an impression otherwise, it rebounds after impression is removed from the mouth unknown to the operator resulting in a tightly fitting crown. It is important that both the syringe low viscosity (LV) or ultralight viscosity (XLV) material and the putty or the heavy viscosity (HV) tray material be flowable at the time of recording the impression.

IMPRESSION TECHNIQUE

Gingival Retraction

There are two techniques of gingival retraction. The double cord and the single cord technique. In the double cord technique, the first cord is placed deep in the sulcus and a second larger cord is packed on top of the first. Before syringing, the top cord is only removed leaving the first cord in the sulcus. The advantage of the double cord is that there is no bleeding or sulcular fluid discharge at the time of impression making because blood, saliva and water can interfere with the flow of the syringe material.[2] If the gingival condition is healthy as seen in the case presented, it is alright to use the single cord technique (Figs. 4.1A to E).

Syringing of Impression Material

Syringing of impression material is started at the bottom of a preparation and circulated around the tooth with the material against the tooth and the syringe tip in the material. Voids occur, if placement is done at different areas, and then brought together. Also care should be taken to see that the material is not pulled away from the tooth. (Figs. 4.1F to H).

"Aquasil" Ultra LV and "Aquasil" Ultra XLV (Dentsply) are flowable materials with thixotropic properties. The material flows well and wets the tooth with a low contact angle when it is syringed, but as soon as you release the pressure on the syringe, the material stays put on the tooth and does not run over the preparations and into the patient's throat as in a maxillary impression. (Fig. 4.1H).

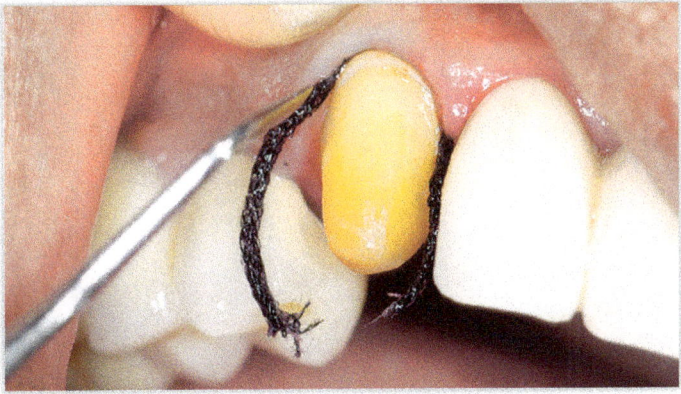

Fig. 4.1A: Packing of cord in progress.

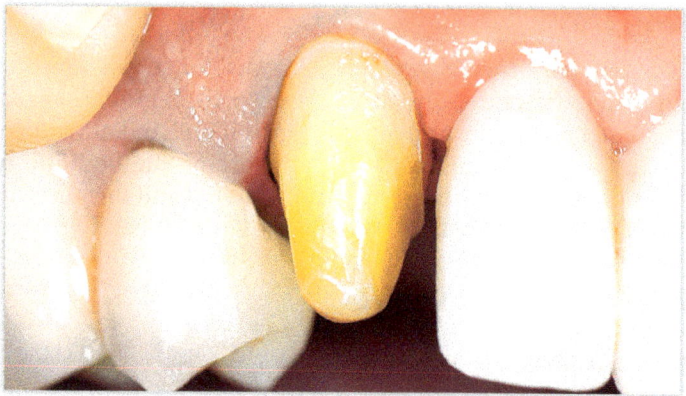

Fig. 4.1B: Completed packing of cord.

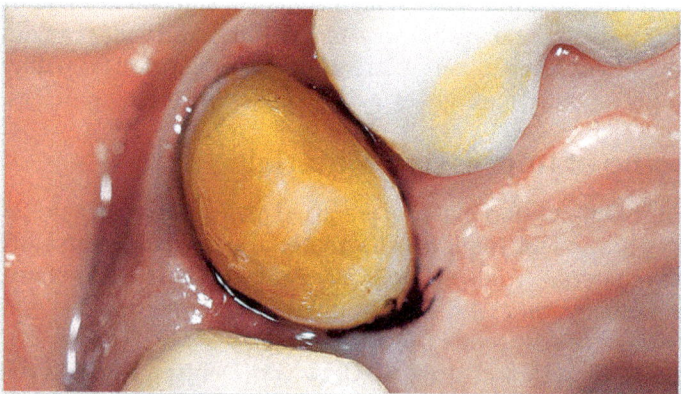

Fig. 4.1C: Occlusal view after completion of packing.

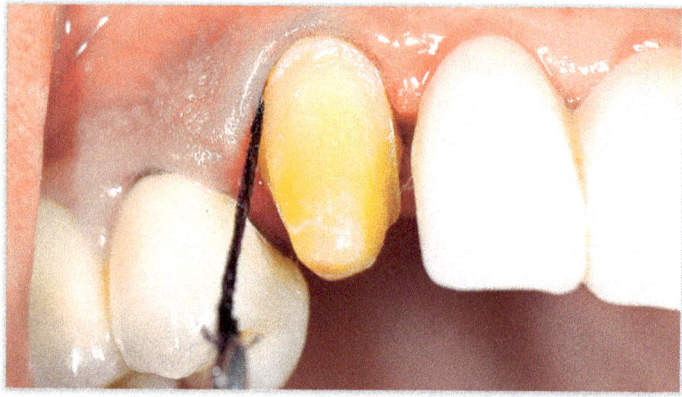

Fig. 4.1D: Removal of cord just prior to impression making.

Impression Making for Implant Supported Prosthesis | 43

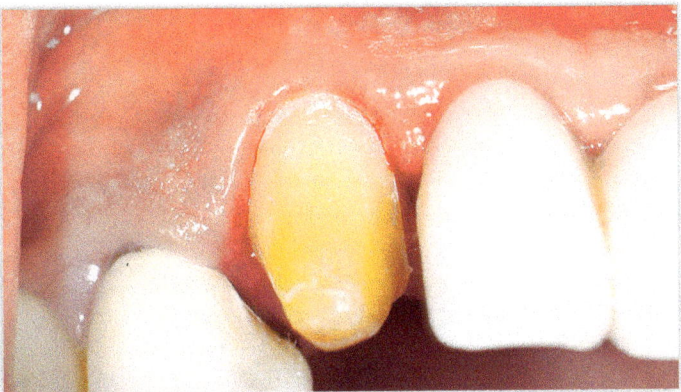

Fig. 4.1E: Observe margins after removal of cord.

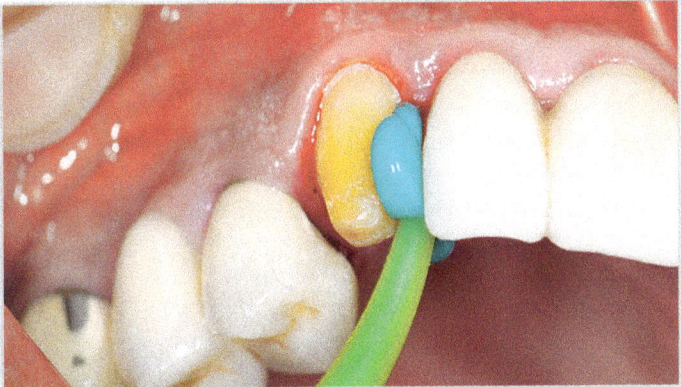

Fig. 4.1F: Initial placement of Aquasil LV keeping syringe tip close to the tooth and at the prepared margin.

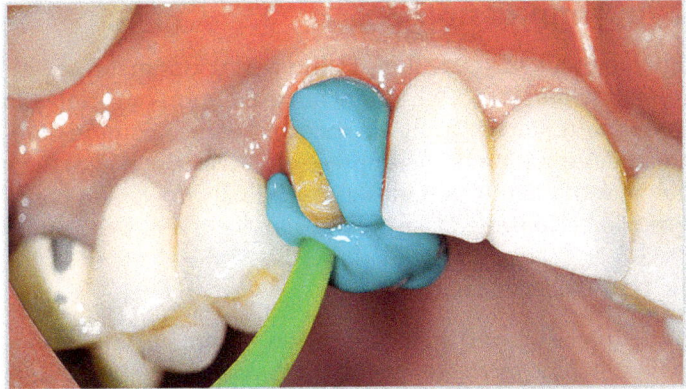

Fig. 4.1G: Observe the syringe tip is in the material and close to the tooth.

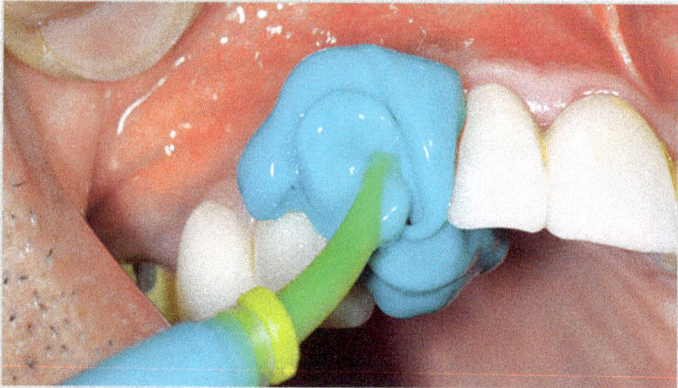

Fig. 4.1H: Completion of the syringing of LV. Observe still the tip is in the material.

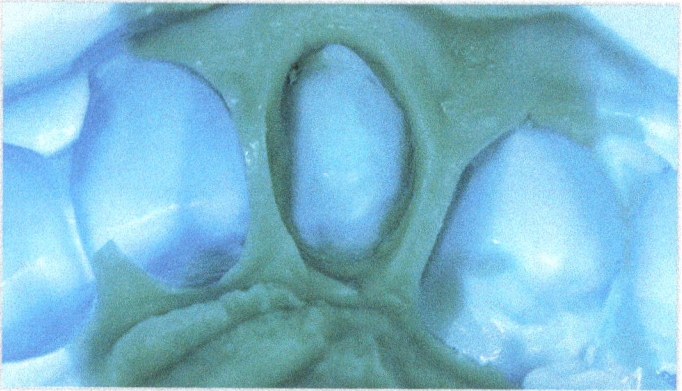

Fig. 4.1I: Observe all the margins recorded in detail. Thin flesh of impression material is observed even beyond the prepared margin. Lingual margin is short of cingulum for the minicrown preparation.

Removing Impression

Although materials such as Aquasil Ultra permit optimal recovery even after compression, generally it is important not to compress an impression material while trying to remove it from the mouth, because compression can cause permanent deformation of the impression. Break the seal of the impression from the back of the tray and loosen it gradually to prevent tears. Only after the impression is loosened, use the tray handle to remove the impression.

Check the Impression

View the impression under magnification for voids, wrinkles and bubbles and to check that no teeth are touching the tray, especially the prepared teeth (Fig. 4.1I). A small bubble or void at the margin is acceptable since the technician will be able to scrape off that bubble without affecting the marginal fit. If however, there is a huge void or overall the impression is not clear and has wrinkles, it is necessary to repeat the impression.

IMPRESSION MAKING FOR IMPLANT SUPPORTED PROSTHESIS

Before undertaking any procedure, an accurate diagnostic wax up by the technician with consultation of the clinician goes a long way in treatment planning and success of final prosthesis (Fig. 4.2A).

The aim of impression making for implant supported prosthesis is to transfer the exact position of the implant in the patient's mouth to that of the laboratory working cast. Different authors have described various techniques for achieving the above but till today there is no consensus on which technique is better than the other. The authors of this paper are of the opinion that whatever method is used, it should be done with the understanding of the technique and the properties of the impression material.

Impression materials should be resilient enough to be removed from undercuts without distortion and at the same time be rigid enough to allow accurate seating of the components and to prevent their movements during pouring of the impression in dental stone.

Although polyethers such as (Impregum, 3M ESPE) have traditionally been used effectively for recording the position of the implant and transferring the same to the working cast, the authors prefer and have vast experience in using a more user-friendly modified crosslinked addition reaction silicone Aquasil Ultra (Dentsply). In order to satisfy the requirements of rigidity and also resilience, the combination of Aquasil Soft Putty and Aquasil Light Viscosity (LV) serves the purpose admirably.

A stock tray is usually sufficient for one or two teeth impressions or for short span bridges. However, for more extensive cases, use the open tray technique by making a custom tray (Fig. 4.2C). For greater accuracy in transferring the position of the implant to the laboratory cast, the open tray technique is recommended by most authorities.[3,4]

In the open tray technique, you have to unscrew the transfer impression copings and subsequently the impression copings are picked up in the impression. This generally is also known as the "Pick up" technique (Figs. 4.2A to L).

In the closed tray technique also known as the "Repositioning technique", the repositioning post remains on the implant after the impression. It is then unscrewed from the implant and repositioned into the accurate putty/light body impression (Figs. 4.3A to D). The implant analog is secured to the repositioning post (Fig. 4.3D) and a gingival remodeling material (Gingival mask) as described above is filled in before making the hard stone cast.

Both the above open and closed tray techniques are implant level impression techniques.

Abutment level impression techniques using the "Snap on" connection are also available with companies such as Straumann ITI (Switzerland), Ankylos Standard (Dentsply, Germany) and 3i Biomet (USA), besides others.

46 Clinical Guide to Oral Implantology: Step by Step Procedures

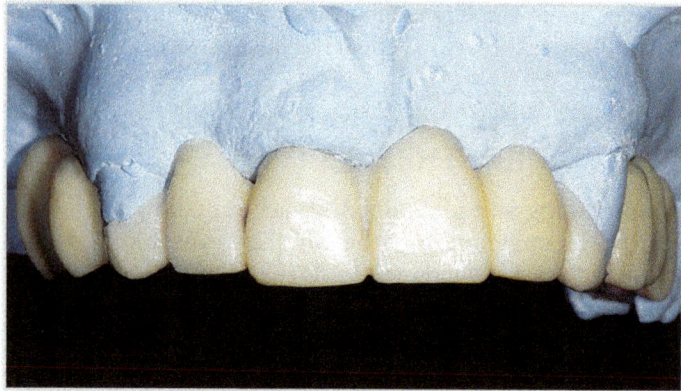

Fig. 4.2A: Wax up done by the technician to aid in planning and to fabricate a surgical stent.

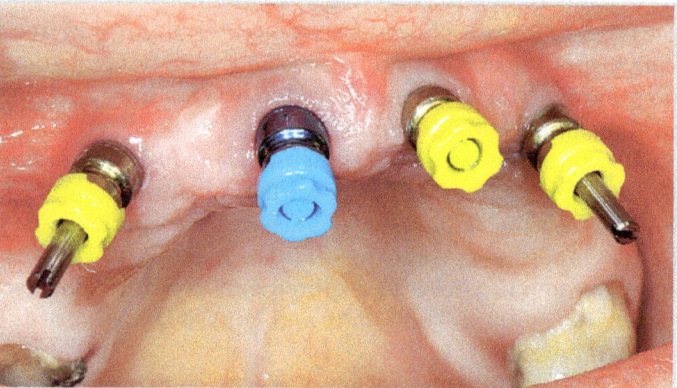

Fig. 4.2B: Combination of open and closed tray technique (Xive implant system, Dentsply Implants, Germany).

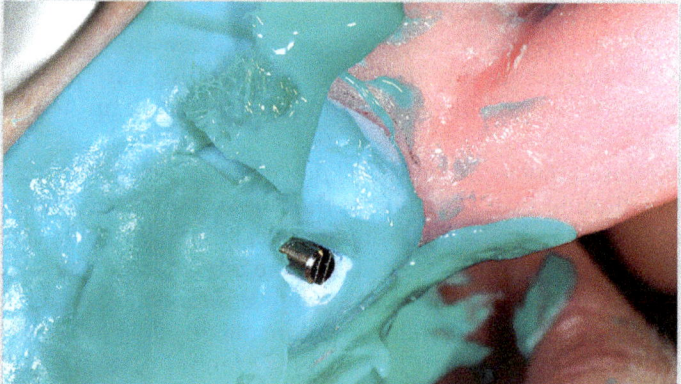

Fig. 4.2C: Open tray technique using custom tray showing the impression post through the impression material.

Impression Making for Implant Supported Prosthesis

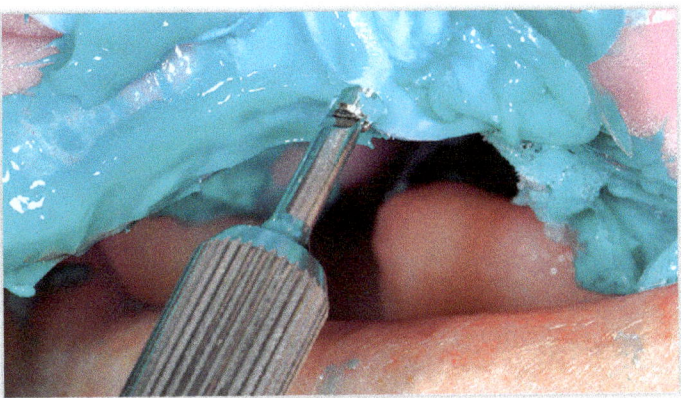

Fig. 4.2D: Unscrewing of the impression post to aid in removal of the impression.

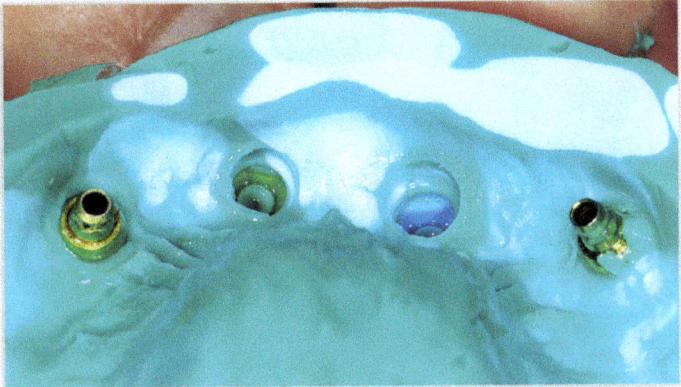

Fig. 4.2E: Impression showing the transfer caps in the center and the transfer copings of the open tray in the canine region.

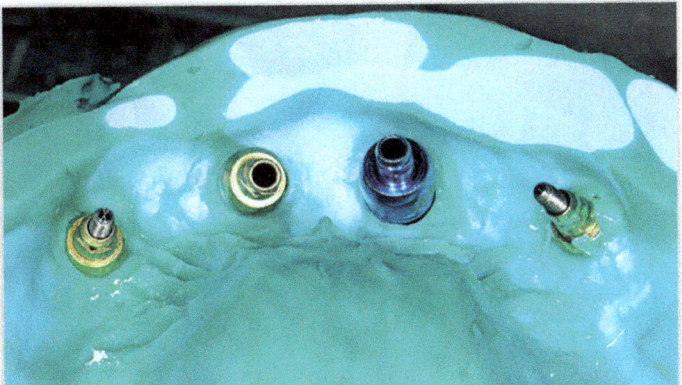

Fig. 4.2F: Impression showing the transfer copings of the closed tray (central incisors) and the open tray transfer copings (canine regions).

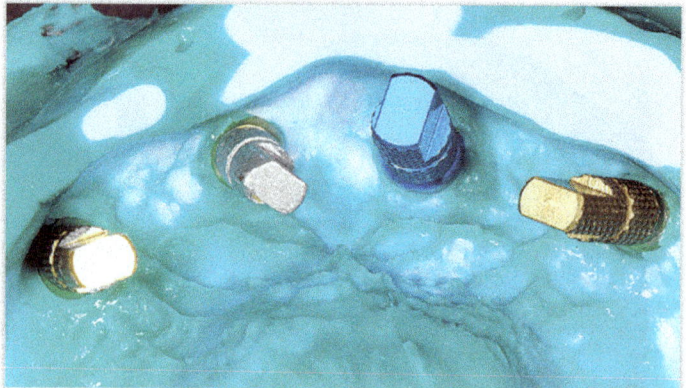

Fig. 4.2G: All four lab analogs screwed into place.

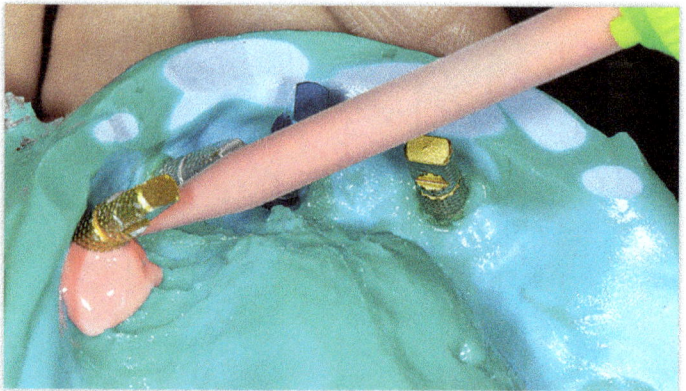

Fig. 4.2H: Gingival mask being poured.

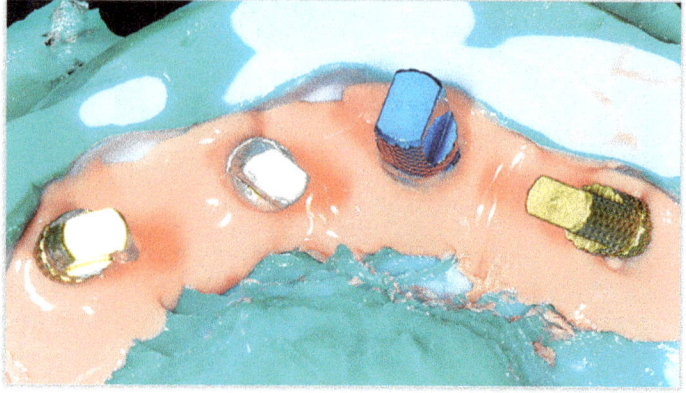

Fig. 4.2I: Gingival mask in place.

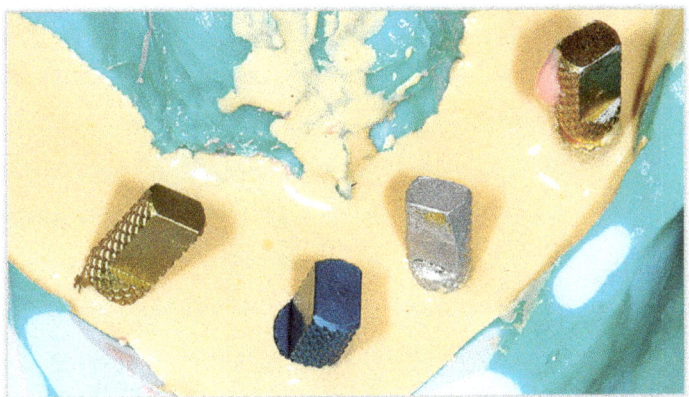

Fig. 4.2J: Die stone poured.

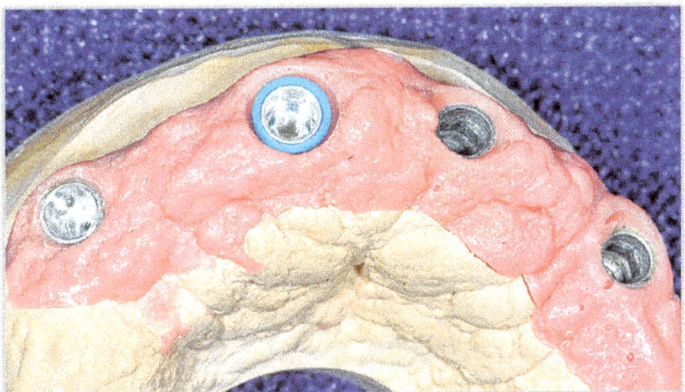

Fig. 4.2K: Cast with the gingival mask and the implant analogs in place, transferring the orientation of the implants (Implant level impression technique).

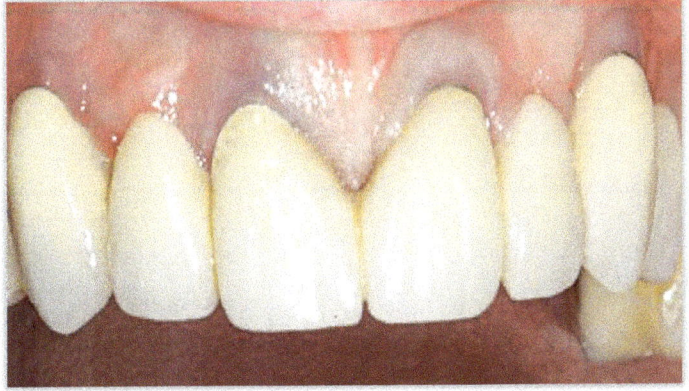

Fig. 4.2L: Final Implant supported PFM fixed prosthesis cemented in patient's mouth.

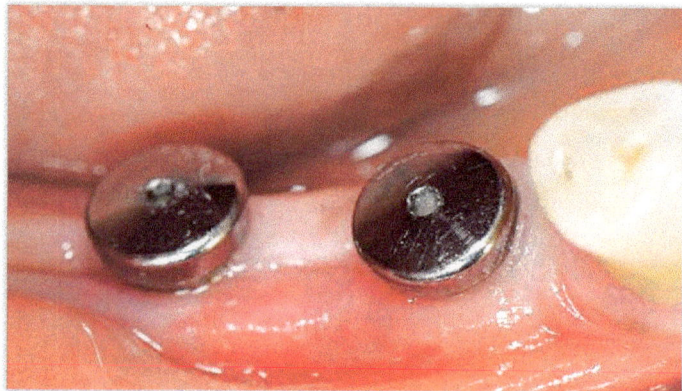

Fig. 4.3A: Ankylos balance sulcus formers in place.

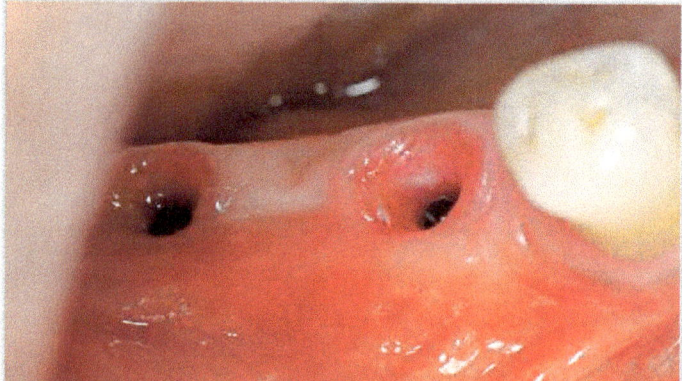

Fig. 4.3B: On removal of the sulcus formers after 10 days, note the excellent healing of the gingiva.

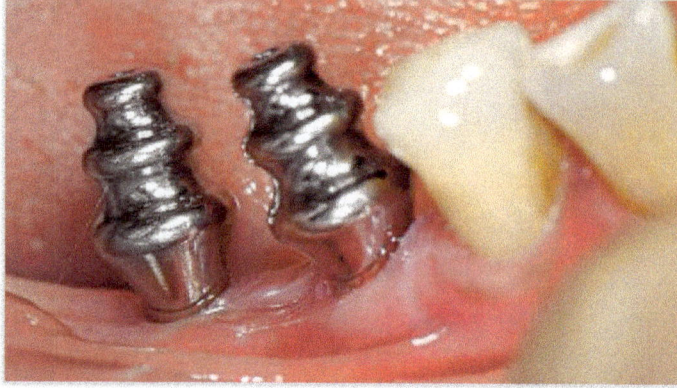

Fig. 4.3C: Repositioning post in place (showing the repositioning technique of impression making).

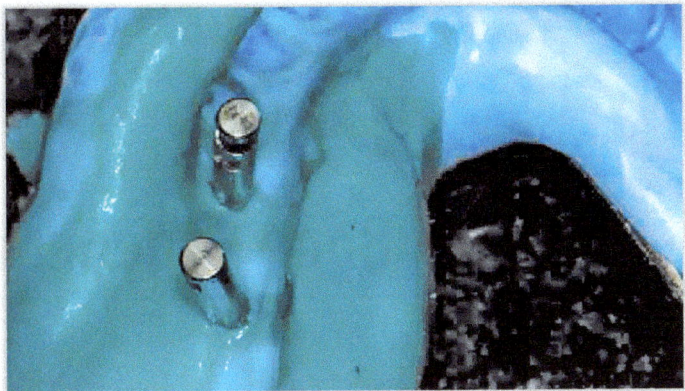

Fig. 4.3D: The transfer posts with implant analogs positioned in Impression (Repositioning Closed tray technique, using Aquasil Putty and LV used in the simultaneous impression technique).

REFERENCES

1. Reality Publishing Co., Vol 22, Texas, 2012;827-32.
2. Nemetz H, Donovan T, Landsman H. Exposing the gingival margin. A systemic approach for the control of haemorrhage, J. Prosthet Dent 1984:51:647-51.
3. Gordon GE, Johnson GH, Drennon DG. The effect of tray selection on the accuracy of elastomeric impression materials. J Prosthet Dent. 1990;63:12-15.
4. Vigolo P, Majzoub Z, Cordioli G. Evaluation of the accurancy of three techniques used for multiple implant abutment impressions. J Prosthet Dent. 2003;89:186-92.

Chapter 5

Bone Regeneration

Loss of alveolar bone due to disease, trauma or surgery can contraindicate the use of dental implants. Bone grafting can provide the functional and structural support in such cases. Grafted bone can be used as a scaffold to regenerate bone lost due to disease, preserve extraction sockets, preserve or augment width and height of alveolar ridges. Autogenous bone remains the gold standard because of its osteogenic and osteoinducing properties which allows bone to form more rapidly. Autogenous block bone grafts are sometimes the only methods of gaining alveolar ridge height.

Allogenic and Xenogenic bone particulates have gained increasing acceptance and popularity as bone regenerative materials in dental implantology. They prove useful in filling in of defects in alveolar ridges, covering exposed implant surfaces and in certain cases (when bone walls are present) in augmenting the width of the alveolar bone before implant placement. Soft tissue ingrowth (epithelium and/or connective tissue) can be a problem with augmentative procedures with any grafting material. Therefore, it is necessary to use non-resorbable or resorbable barrier membranes which are cell occlusive and prevent epithelial and connective tissue cells from ingrowing in the defect. This technique of allowing bone to grow by osteoconduction and/or osteoinduction, and preventing soft tissue growth by barrier membranes is called *guided bone regeneration* (GBR) (Fig. 5.1).

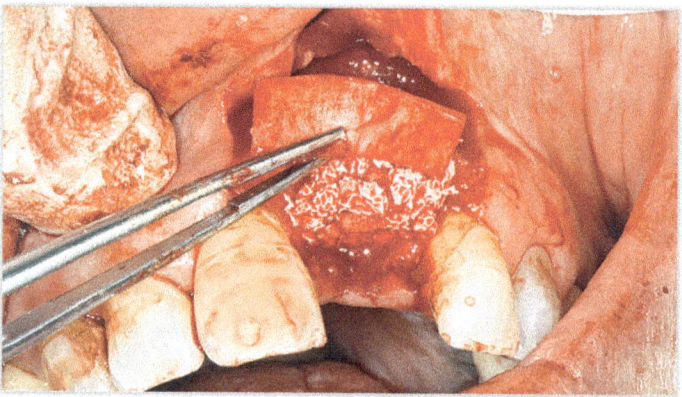

Fig. 5.1: Barrier membrane placed over bone substitute.

It is important to differentiate between osteoinduction and osteoconduction. Autogenous bone, i.e. bone harvested from the same individual is osteoinductive meaning it is capable of forming new bone without the presence of any bony walls. Whereas allogenic (human), xenogenic (animal) or alloplastic (synthetic) bone are osteoconductive and require the presence of bony walls to form new natural bone. They cannot form new bone by themselves when placed in soft tissues. The most commonly used method of bone reformation in everyday implantology practice is by GBR. The open trabecular structures of bone substitutes provide an environment of revascularization from the remaining bony walls. Osteogenic progenitor cells from the bloodstream next differentiate into osteoblasts which layers new bone around the graft trabeculae, while the osteoclasts simultaneously resorb the entrapped synthetic bone until they are partially or completely replaced by new bone. The process is known as 'creeping substitution'. This requires about 4-6 months for completion.

BONE SUBSTITUTES

Allogenic Bone

Allogenic bone is usually obtained from human cadavers who have donated their bodies. The most commonly used forms are freeze dried, solvent preserved or irradiated to reduce its antigenicity. Freeze dried bone allografts (FDBA) can be either mineralized or demineralized (DFDBA), generally mineralized freeze-dried bone allograft (MFDBA) is preferred.

Solvent Preserved Allogenic Bone

Puros (Zimmer Dental, USA) is solvent preserved as opposed to freeze drying to extract the water content. Animal and human studies of this material have been shown to produce good bone formation and repair results.

Irradiated Allogenic Bone

Irradiated cancellous bone (Rocky Mountain Tissue Bank, USA) has also been used and recommended as a bone substitute for autogenous bone. Unfortunately, it has lack of published scientific documentation.

Alloplastic Bone Substitutes

Alloplasts are not natural components of bone materials. They are either bioactive glass (Perioglass, USA), beta-tricalcium Phosphate (beta-TCP), Cerasorb (Curasan, Germany) or Calcium Sulphate. Documented alloplastic grafting materials are beta-TCP, Cerasorb, Curasan, Germany.

Tricalcium Phosphates

Cerasorb (Curasan, Germany) is beta-tricalcium phosphate. The material is resorbed completely and replaced by new bone in a period of 3 to 4 months. It is recommended for use in all grafting procedures. However, in more demanding ridge morphologies such as lateral augmentation, the resorption rate of beta-

TCP is too high to allow time for new bone formation. Therefore, recently a few companies have added hydroxyapatite (HA) in a ratio of 30:70 to reduce the resorption rate.

Algae-derived Bone Substitute (DentsplySirona Implants, Germany)

Frios Algipore is an inorganic component of a certain red algae. The basic scaffold possesses an interconnecting network porous microstructure. Frios Algipore has been in clinical use for over 20 years and has been documented as an augmentation material in numerous clinical studies;[1,2] Algipore is largely resorbed and replaced by new bone by the process of remodeling. It is widely used in all grafting procedures including sinus grafting.

Chemically and Thermally Treated Xenogenic Bone Grafts

The most popular and time tested (animal and human studies) bovine bone substitutes is Bio-Oss (Geistlich, Switzerland).[3-5] It is inorganic bovine bone that has been chemically and thermally treated to remove its organic component. Bio-Oss is osteoconductive and over time the graft undergoes physiologic remodeling and becomes incorporated with the surrounding bone. Bio-Oss has been successfully used in a number of clinical situations including intrabony defects, maxillary sinus augmentations, GBR and around implants.

It can also be mixed with autogenous bone in a ratio of 80% Bio-Oss, 20% autogenous bone for faster bone regeneration. Bio-Oss can be used alone or with barrier membranes.

Since the GBR technique has become the standard of care in daily practice, case reports with the technique and materials preferred by the authors will be described. The authors prefer to use Bio-Oss (Geistlich, Switzerland) and a non-crosslinked resorbable membrane Bio-Gide (Geistlich, Switzerland). A resorbable membrane such as Bio-Gide offers several advantages over non-resorbable ones, like easy clinical handling during surgery due to its hydrophilic properties, low risk of complications arising in cases where soft tissue exposures take place, no need of a second surgical intervention for membrane removal. However, these resorbable membranes tend to collapse and have a rather short barrier function. For these disadvantages, the authors prefer to combine collagen membranes with appropriate bone substitutes such as Bio-Oss (Geistlich, Switzerland) frequently mixed with autogenous bonechips locally harvested with bone scrapers.

CASE 1

Guided Bone Regeneration (GBR) Followed by Implant Placement

Female-aged 70 years reports with pain and swelling in upper left central incisor. Radiological examination indicates the possibility of a vertical root fracture (Fig. 5.2A). It was therefore decided to extract the tooth and replace it with an implant. On extraction of the tooth, it was revealed that there was complete loss of buccal plate of bone right upto the apex of the tooth. It was therefore decided to not resort to immediate implantation but do GBR in a staged procedure for implant placement. Two vertical releasing incisions were taken (Fig. 5.2B). Reflection of a full thickness mucoperiosteal flap revealed extensive loss of bone buccally and mesiodistally (Fig. 5.2B). It was therefore decided to harvest bone from the nasal spine to take advantage of the osteogenic and osteoinductive properties of autogenous bone (Fig. 5.3). Looking to the extensive regeneration of bone required, it was decided to tack the collagen membrane, thus ensuring greater stability of the same (Fig. 5.4). Autogenous bone from the nasal spine was particulated and mixed with Bio-Oss particles covering the defect area and also over-contouring the same (Fig. 5.5). Primary closure was obtained by releasing the periosteal flap at the apex with a new No. 15 blade. After a period of 6 months excellent regeneration of the ridge was observed (Fig. 5.6). An Ankylos B/14 Implant was placed in the correct 3-D position (Fig. 5.7). Abutment was placed and provisionalized with composite crown on the same day (Fig. 5.8).

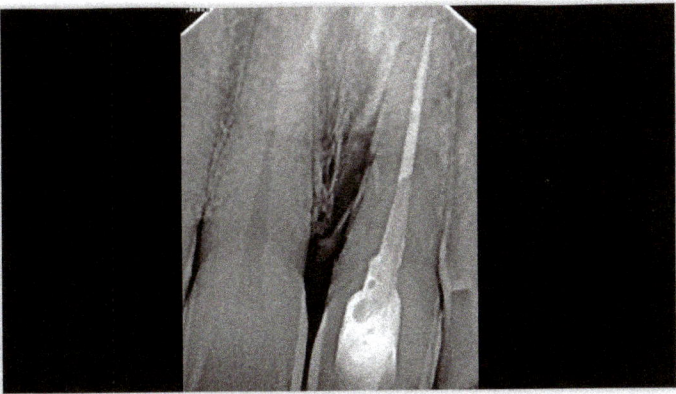

Fig. 5.2A: Intraoral periapical (IOPA) showing vertical root fracture.

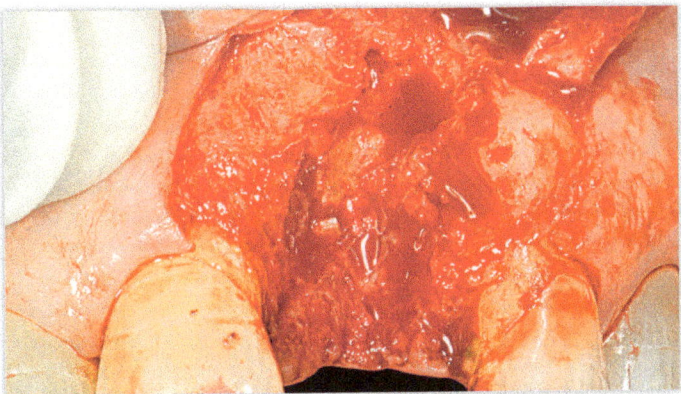

Fig. 5.2B: Large bony defect making implant placement impossible.

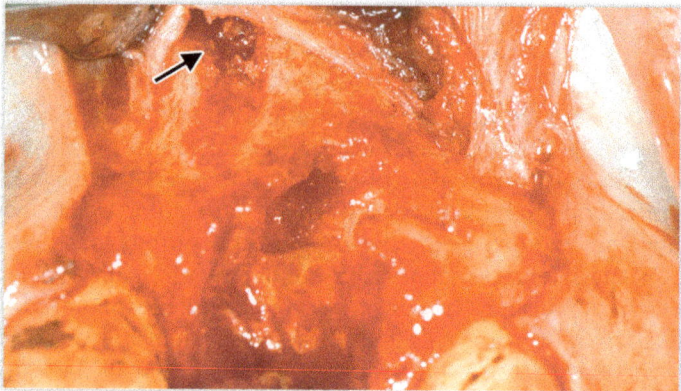

Fig. 5.3: Harvesting of bone from nasal spine.

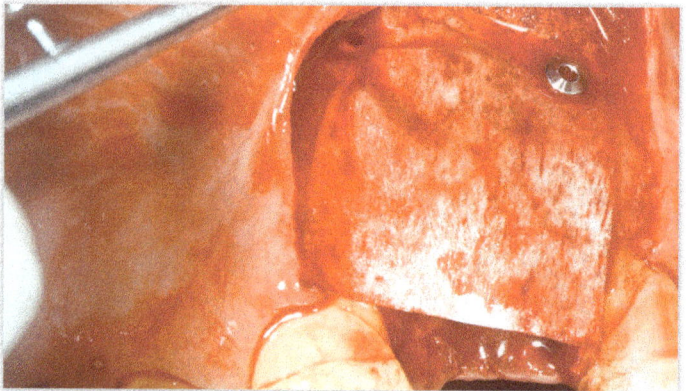

Fig. 5.4: Bio-Gide collagen membrane stabilized with tacking pins.

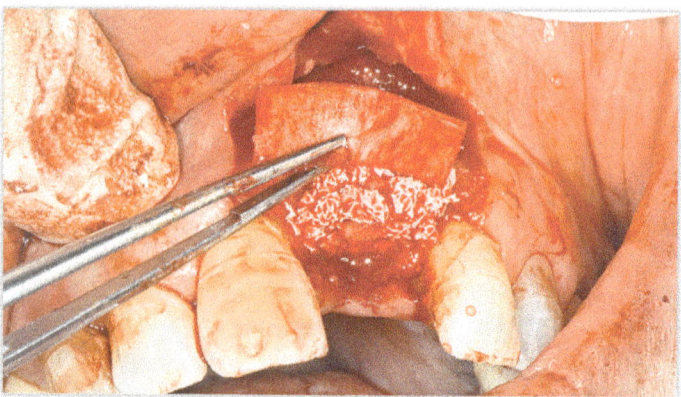

Fig. 5.5: Autogenous bone mixed with Bio-Oss particles is covered with stabilized collagen membrane.

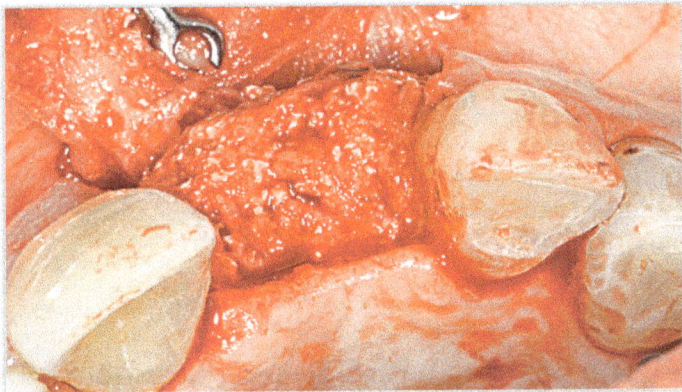

Fig. 5.6: Excellent regeneration of new bone after 6 months.

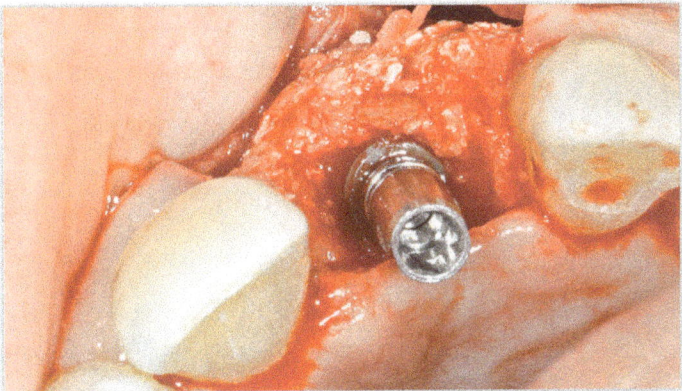

Fig. 5.7: Correct three-dimensional placement of implant in grafted bone.

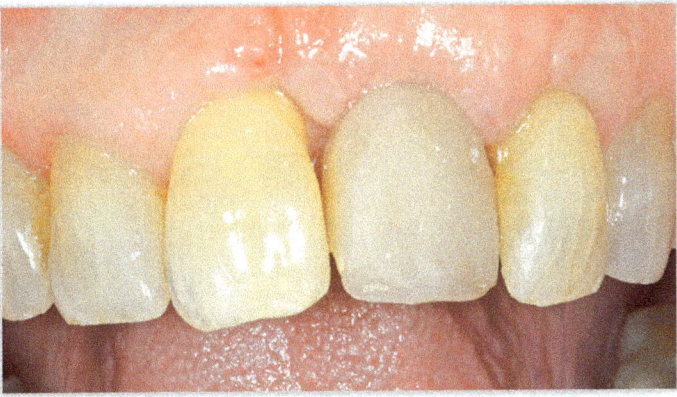

Fig. 5.8: Provisional composite restoration placed immediately after second stage surgery. Tissues will be allowed to stabilize for three months before definitive restoration.

After a period of 2 months of waiting for the soft tissues to stabilize a crown and bridge impression was taken and a layered Zircornia crown was given for fabrication. The crown was cemented with a definitive cement and placement of retraction cord (Fig. 5.9). The placement of retraction cords in the sulcus before final cementing aids in removal of the cement subgingivally. Thus helps in preventing cement related peri-implantitis (Fig.5.10). The two year follow-up picture shows healthy peri-impant tissues and spontaneous regeneration of interdental papilla (Fig 5.11).

CASE 2

Block Bone Grafting with Delayed Placement of Implant

Female aged 25 years has old failing Porcelain Fused to Metal (PFM) bridge replacing two upper central incisors with lateral incisors as abutments. The lateral incisors have been endodontically treated. Looking to the young age

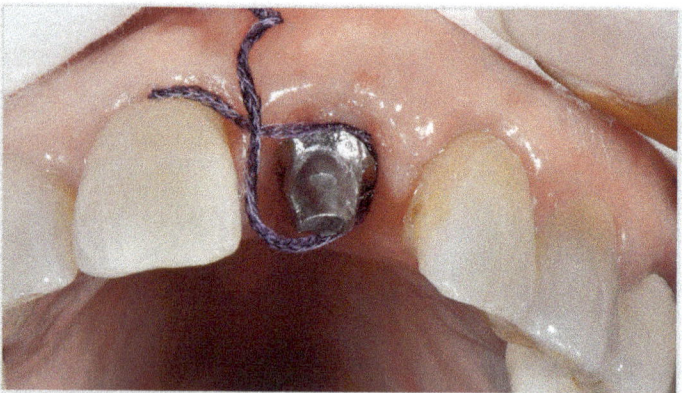

Fig. 5.9: Retraction cord (#000) placed before taking final impression.

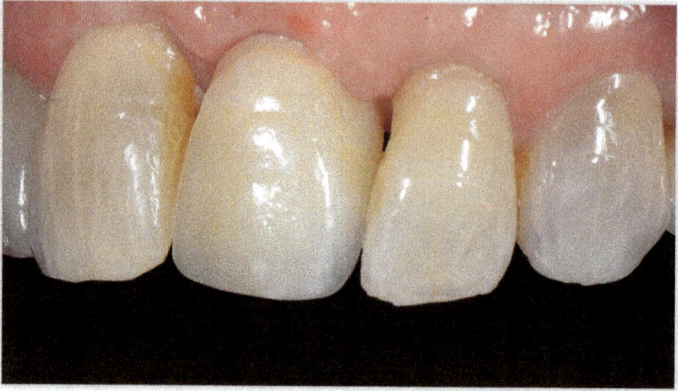

Fig. 5.10: Crown (21) immediately after cementation. Note absence of interdental papilla.

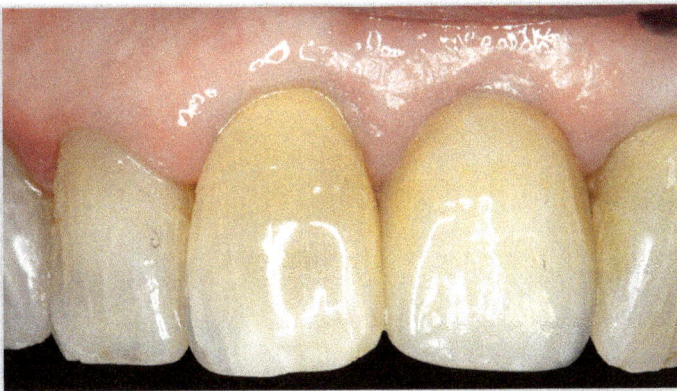

Fig. 5.11: Two-year follow-up showing spontaneous regeneration of the papillae.

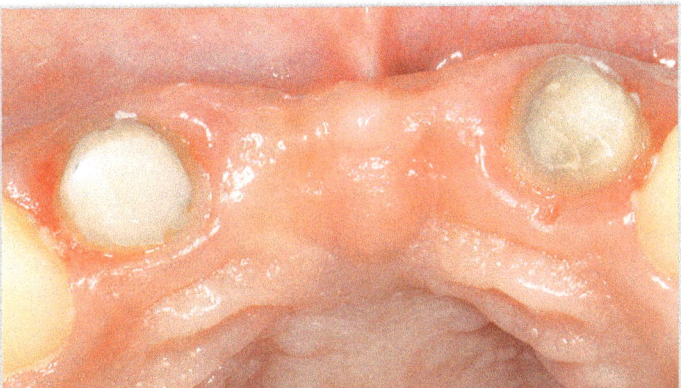

Fig. 5.12: Lateral incisor are weak abutments for fixed partial denture (FPD).

of the patient and the poor prognosis of the lateral incisors as abutments, it was decided to place a single implant in the upper right central incisor with a cantilever pontic and place two single crowns on the lateral incisors, thus taking the load away from the weak lateral incisors (Fig. 5.12).

Preoperative Evaluation

Ridge mapping and CBCT evaluation confirmed the narrow width of the ridge to place even the smallest diameter of the implant. Since this basically would be a one wall defect, it was decided to do block bone grafting instead of guided bone regeneration because of greater predictability (Fig. 5.13).

Operative Procedures

A block of bone from the retromolar area was harvested using Piezosurgery (Acteon, India) (Fig. 5.14). The block bone was rigidly fixated to the decorticated host bone using a single screw using the Ustomed kit (Ustomed, Germany) (Fig. 5.15).

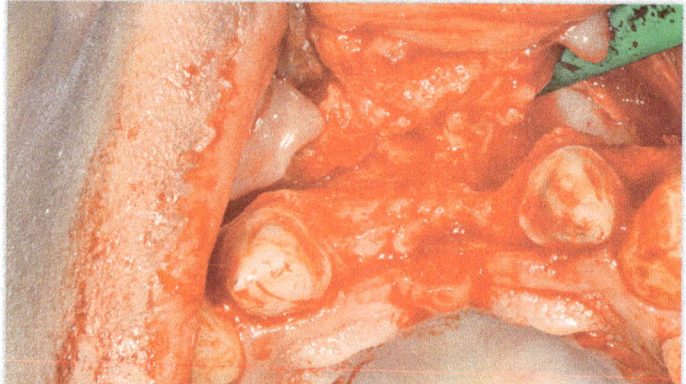

Fig. 5.13: The ridge is too thin to support any width of implants.

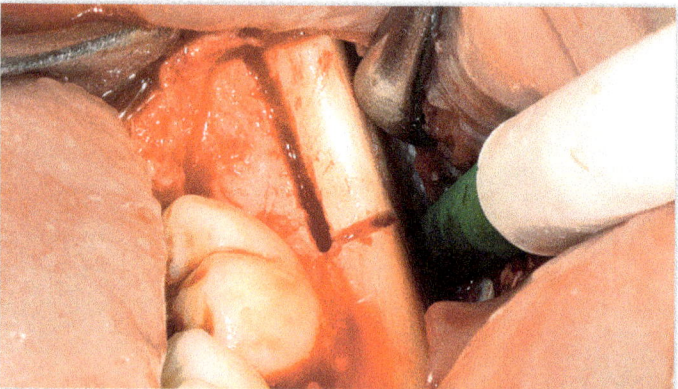

Fig. 5.14: Harvesting of block bone from retromolar area using piezosurgery.

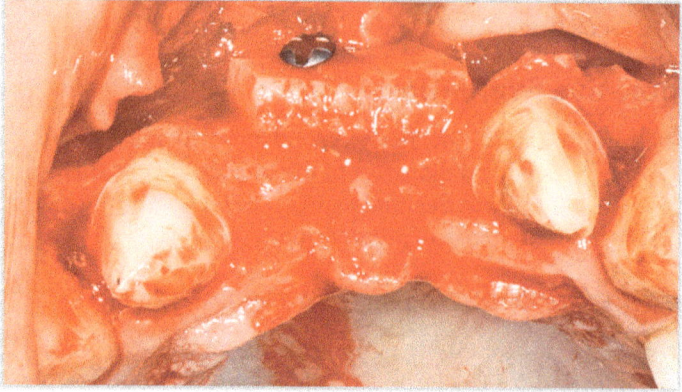

Fig. 5.15: Block bone graft secured firmly with only one osteosynthesis screw.

For greater predictability and to prevent the block bone from resorbing it was decided to combine block bone grafting with guided bone regeneration (GBR) (Figs. 5.16 and 5.17). After waiting for a period of 5 months Ankylos implant of diameter 3.5 mm and length of 14 mm was placed (Figs. 5.18 and 5.19). After waiting for a further period of 3 months an abutment was torqued in at 15 N cm (Fig. 5.20). The tissues were allowed to stabilize for a further period of 2 months during which time she was rehabilitated with provisional crowns on the lateral incisors and a cantilever bridge on the implant.

The final restorations were fabricated in lithium disilicate (Emax Ivoclar, India) (Fig. 5.21).

CASE 3

Guided Bone Regeneration Using Autogenous Bone, Layered with Bone Substitute

Male aged 34 years comes with the chief complaint of pain and swelling around his old fixed partial denture. Cone beam CT and radiological examination reveals external root resorption and infection due to tooth 21 (Fig. 5.22). The patient requested extraction and immediate implantation due to lack of time as he lives abroad. Extraction of tooth 21 revealed both horizontal and vertical loss of bone which necessitated grafting of autogenous bone because of its proven osteogenic, osteoinductive and osteoconductive properties.

Bone was harvested from the retromolar area making 3 Audi rings with a 7 mm trephine bur (Fig. 5.23). The bone was particulated with the help of a bone cruncher (Fig. 5.24). Ankylos implant after placement revealed exposure of 3 threads and collar of the implant (Fig. 5.25). The particulated autogenous bone was directly placed all around the exposed implant as the first layer (Fig. 5.26).

For contour augmentation and to prevent the autogenous bone from resorbing the same was covered with small particle size Bio-Oss

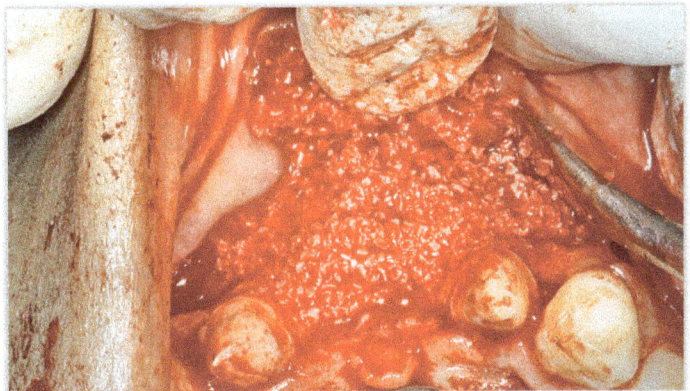

Fig. 5.16: Deficiencies between block bone and recipient site was filled with bone substitutes. Also the block bone was covered.

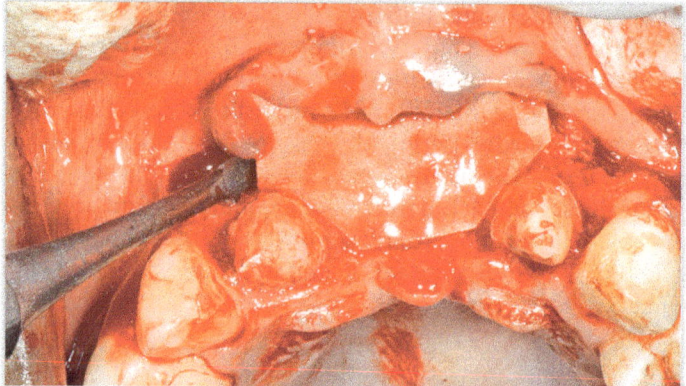

Fig. 5.17: Collagen membrane placed over grafted area to prevent soft tissue infiltration.

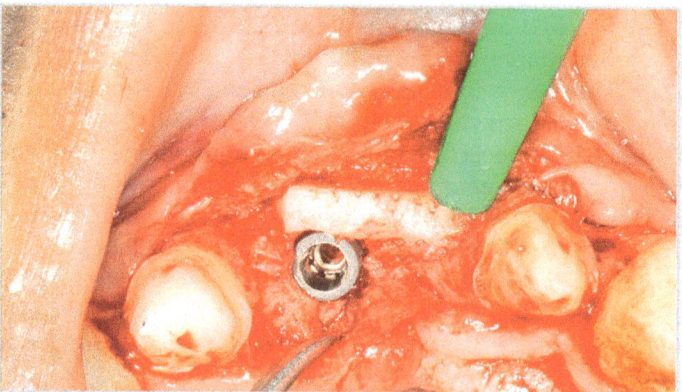

Fig. 5.18: Ankylos implant in place.

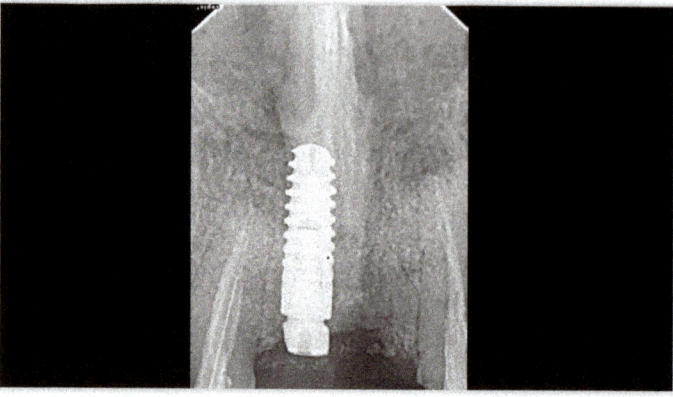

Fig. 5.19: IOPA after placement of implant.

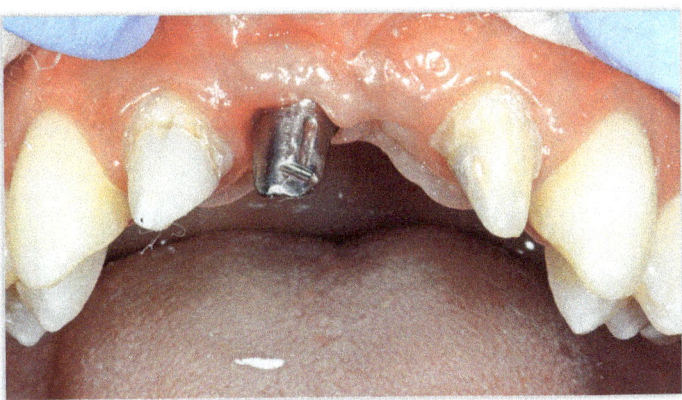

Fig. 5.20: Abutment torqued into place.

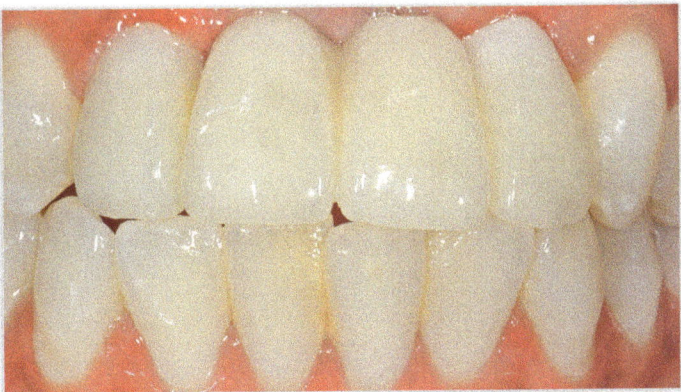

Fig. 5.21: Single all ceramic crowns on lateral incisors and implant supported cantilever bridge on right central incisor.

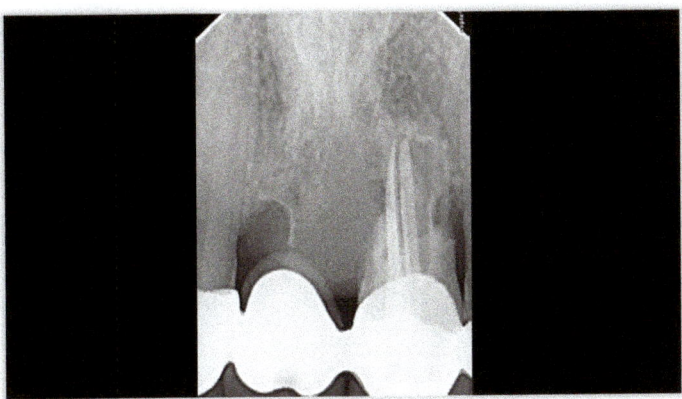

Fig. 5.22: Preoperative IOPA showing extensive external root resorption of 21.

64 Clinical Guide to Oral Implantology: Step by Step Procedures

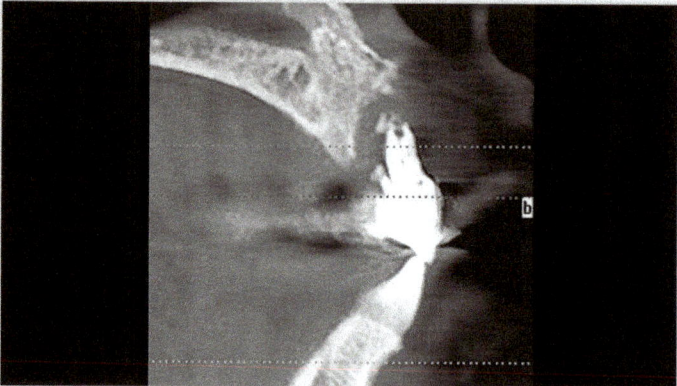

Fig. 5.23: CBCT picture showing complete loss of labial as well as palatal alveolar bone.

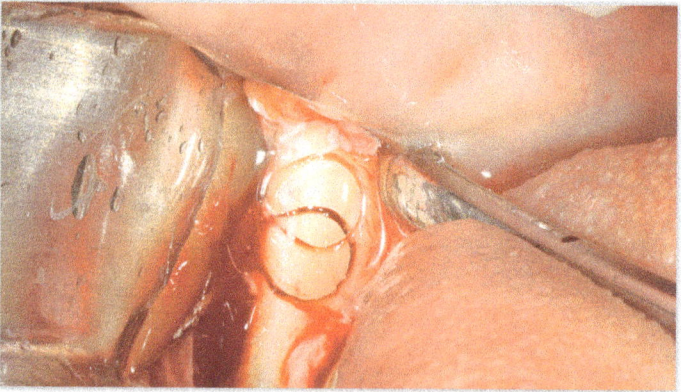

Fig. 5.24: Audi rings made at the retromolar area with the help of trephine burs.

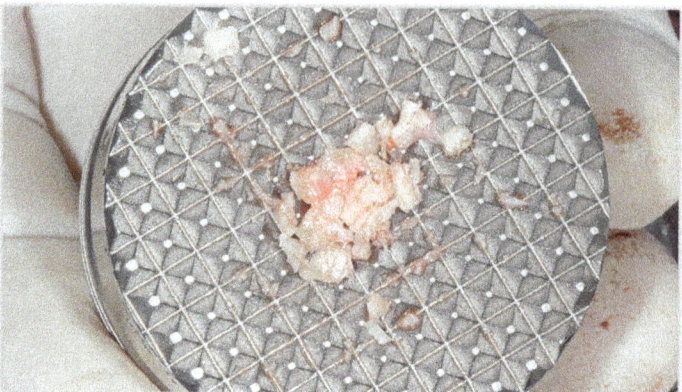

Fig. 5.25: Harvested bone particulated with a bone cruncher.

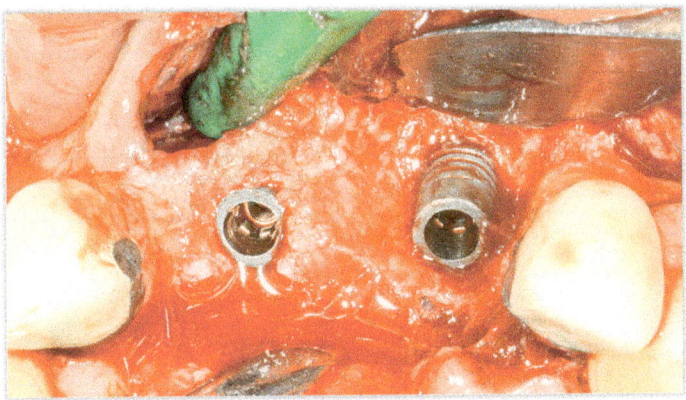

Fig. 5.26: Implant in 21 region shows no bone coverage 360° in the coronal part of the implant.

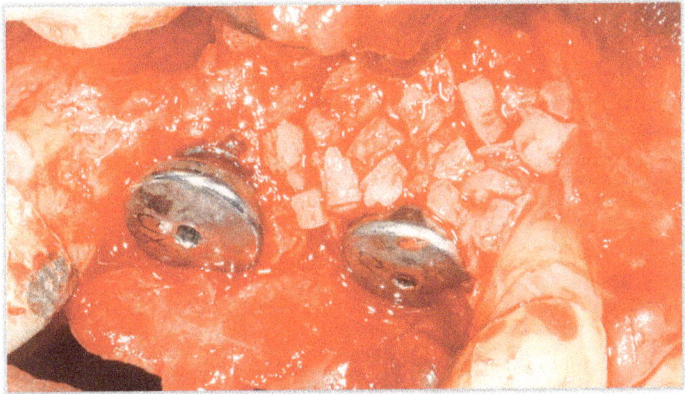

Fig. 5.27: Particulated autogenous bone placed as the first layer covering the exposed part of the implant.

(Geistlich, Germany). To prevent soft tissue infiltration into the grafted site a wel-documented cell occlusive resorbable collagen membrane "Bio-Gide" (Geistlich, Switzerland) was used. After a healing period of 5 months, Ankylos balance abutments were torqued in with the help of transfer resin jigs. Crown and Bridge impression of the abutments and adjacent lateral incisors were taken to fabricate lithium disilicate all ceramic crowns (Emax Press, Ivoclar Lichtenstein) (Figs. 5.27 to 5.32).

CBCT image after regeneration shows excellent regeneration of lost horizontal and vertical bone height (Fig. 5.33).

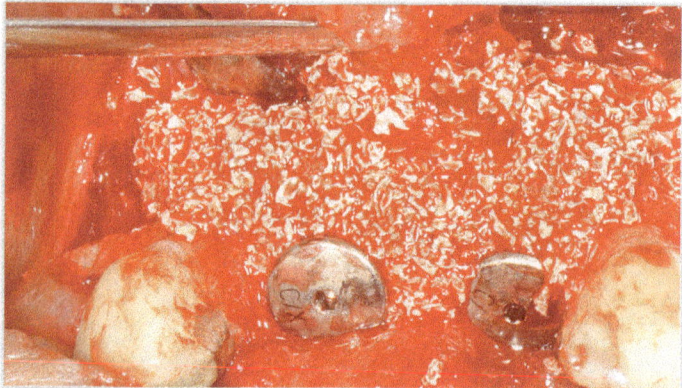

Fig. 5.28: Slow-resorbing Bio-Oss covering the autogenous bone as well as remaining part of the labial ridge for contour augmentation and prevention of resorption of autogenous bone.

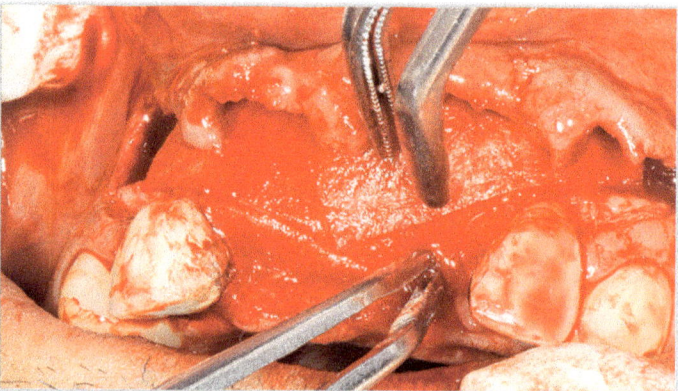

Fig. 5.29: Resorbable collagen membrane Bio-Gide stabilizes the grafted bone and prevents soft tissue migration into the defect area.

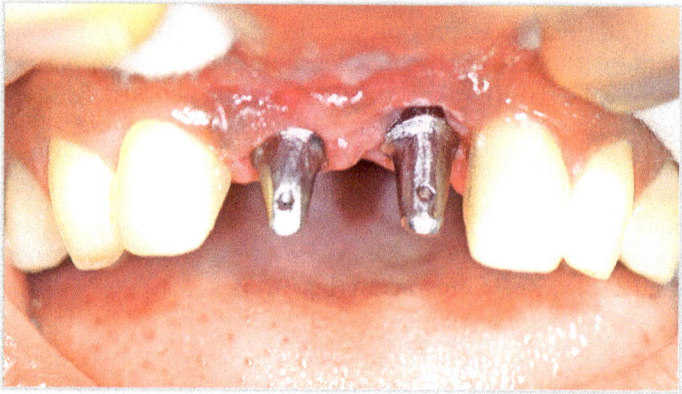

Fig. 5.30: Abutment torqued in with the help of resin transfer jig.

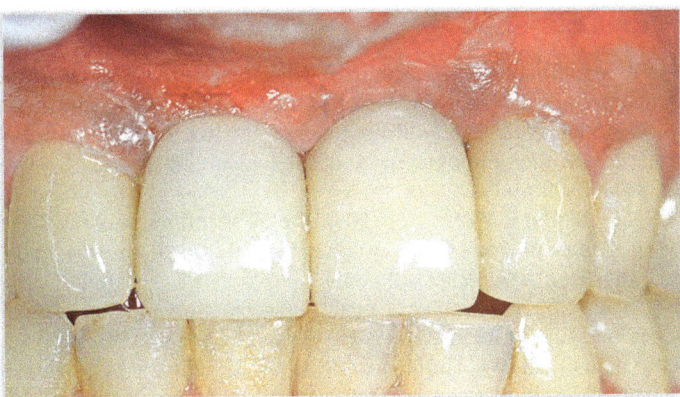

Fig. 5.31: Lithium disilicate crowns after cementation.

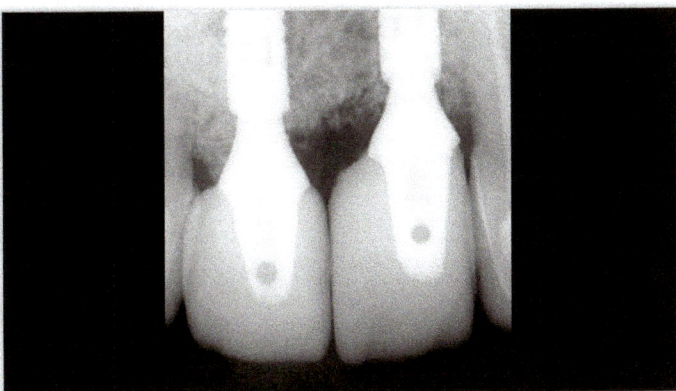

Fig. 5.32: Excellent marginal fit of all ceramic crowns.

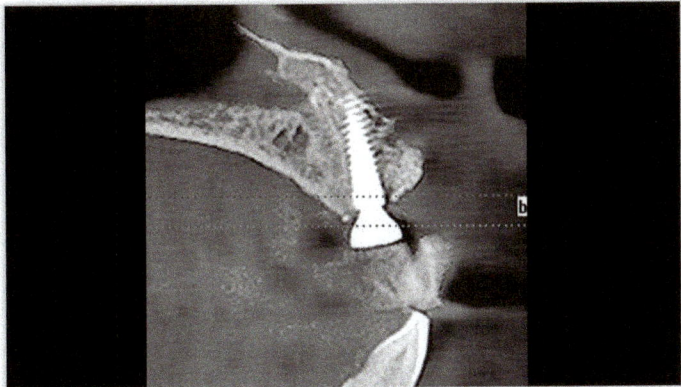

Fig. 5.33: CBCT image after treatment with healing period of 6 months. Note the excellent regeneration of lost horizontal and vertical height.

REFERENCES

1. Ewers R. Maxilla sinus grafting with marine algae derived bone-forming material: a clinical report of long-term results. J Oral Maxillofac Surg. 2005;63(12):1712-23.
2. Thorwarth M, Wehrhan F, Srour S, et al. Evaluation of substitutes for bone: comparison of microradiographic and histological assessments. Br J Oral Maxillofac Surg. 2007;45(1):41-7.
3. Araújo M1, Linder E, Wennström J, Lindhe J. The influence of Bio-Oss Collagen on healing of an extraction socket: an experimental study in the dog. Int J Periodontics Restorative Dent. 2008;28(2):123-35.
4. Jensen SS, Aaboe M, Pinholt EM, et al. Tissue reaction and material characteristics of four bone substitutes. Int J Oral Maxillofac Implants. 1996;11(1):55-66.
5. Norton MR, Odell EW, Thompson ID, Cook RJ. Efficacy of bovine bone mineral for alveolar augmentation: a human histologic study. Clin Oral Implants Res. 2003;14(6):775-83.

Chapter 6

Sinus Grafting

RECONSTRUCTION OF THE ATROPHIC POSTERIOR MAXILLA

Introduction

The maxillary posterior edentulous situation presents many unique problems in rehabilitation with implants. The available alveolar bone height is lost in the posterior maxilla due to periodontal disease before teeth loss and after teeth loss due to pneumatization of the sinus cavity. Therefore, there is dual resorption from the crest of the ridge and from expansion of the sinus cavity. Implants in the posterior maxilla of a height less than 9 mm have been reported to have a lower success rate. The limited height in the posterior maxilla is compounded by bone with poor density as also decrease in bone width. Grafting of the maxillary sinus to overcome the problem of reduced vertical bone height has become a predictable procedure since the 1980's. Studies have reported success rates of over 90% with sinus grafting. Tatum[1] and later on Boyne and James[2] have been credited as the pioneers in sinus grafting procedures.

There are basically two methods of elevating the membrane from the sinus floor in order to place implants of sufficient height. The first one is the osteotome technique which uses a crestal approach through the prepared osteotomy and the other is the lateral sinus window technique. The authors prefer to use the osteotome technique when at least 5 mm of bone height is available from the crest to the floor of the sinus. By careful use of the implant drills, osteotomes or piezosurgery is used to raise the sinus floor 4-5 mm without perforating the membrane.

Surgical Technique for Lifting the Sinus Membrane with Osteotomes (Crestal Approach)

The osteotomy is made 1 mm short of the floor of the sinus using conventional osteotomy drills of the Ankylos system in bone of good density (Fig. 6.1). In poor quality bone after the initial Lindemann drill, bone condensers are used to condense the bone instead of drilling it away (MIS Implants). These condensers have a pointed tip which can prepare an osteotomy in poor quality

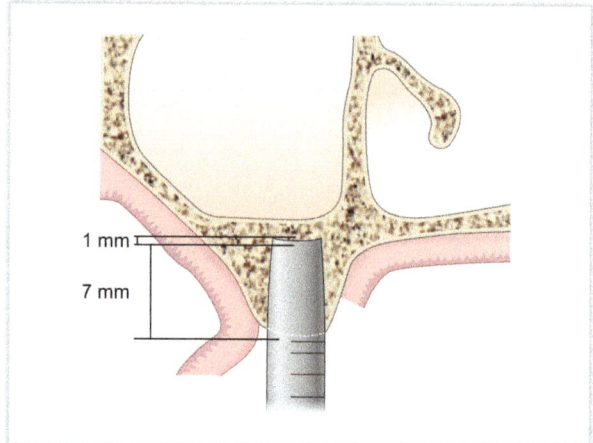

Fig. 6.1: Osteotome at the floor of the sinus.

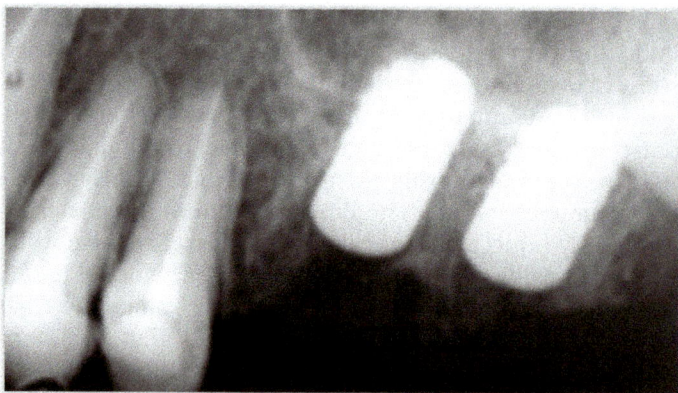

Fig. 6.2: Implants placed through the sinus floor and tenting the sinus membrane.

bone. However, the actual fracture of the floor of the sinus is done with the concave tip osteotomes.

A mallet is used with the osteotome to create a fracture of the floor of the sinus. Careful observation of the markings on the osteotome coupled with listening to a duller sound when osteotome fractures the sinus floor. The osteotome is then removed and the patient is asked to exhale through the nose with the nares pinched. Any perforation can be detected with the expiration of the air through the osteotomy. The instrument is then gently inserted deeper to the desired height and the integrity of the sinus is again confirmed. In most cases, there is no need to tap the bone. Place the implant very slowly to the required depth (Fig. 6.2). Since there is no way to ascertain that at this stage, i.e. while placing the implant the sinus membranes could have perforated the authors recommend not to place any grafting material. Reports have indicated that just the tenting of the membrane with the implant can induce bone formation around it.[3-5]

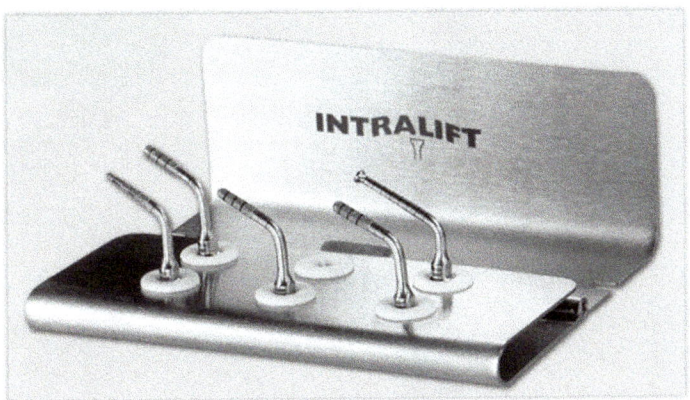

Fig. 6.3: Acteon Intralift kit.

Surgical Technique, of Raising the Sinus Membrane with Piezosurgery (Crestal Approach)

In this technique conventional 2 mm drill of the Ankylos system is used to prepare the Osteotomy 1 to 2 mm short of the sinus floor. The authors prefer to use the Piezosurgery by Acteon (France) namely their Intra lift kit. There are four tips available for Osteotomy) preparation namely, TKW1 1.6 mm, TKW2 2.1 mm, TKW3 2.35 mm and TKW4 2.8 mm (Fig. 6.3).

With each tip floor of the sinus is broken carefully without penetrating too deeply. After the final 3 mm TKW4 tip you may use TKW5 tip to further raise the Schneiderian membrane by hydrodynamic pressure. The Ankylos 3.5 mm or the Xive 3.4 mm (Dentsply Sirona) implant is now placed without any further manipulation of the osteotomy site.

Surgical Approach for Lifting the Sinus Membrane Through Lateral Sinus Window

In the past available host bone measurements with less than 5 mm in height was deemed inadequate to maintain primary stability of an endosteal implant in the sinus cavity. Thus, in these cases simultaneous bone grafting and implant placement was contraindicated in favor of the 2 step approach in which implant placement is delayed until 6 months after the grafting. In recent years, this concept has been challenged with workers reporting success with as little as 1-2 mm of crestal bone available in height. However, adequate ridge width should be available for implant placement.

Anesthesia

Infiltration anaesthesia has been proved to be useful for sinus graft surgery.

Incision and Reflection

A crestal incision is made slightly on the palatal aspect of the edentulous ridge (Fig. 6.4). This incision is made taking awareness of the greater palatine artery

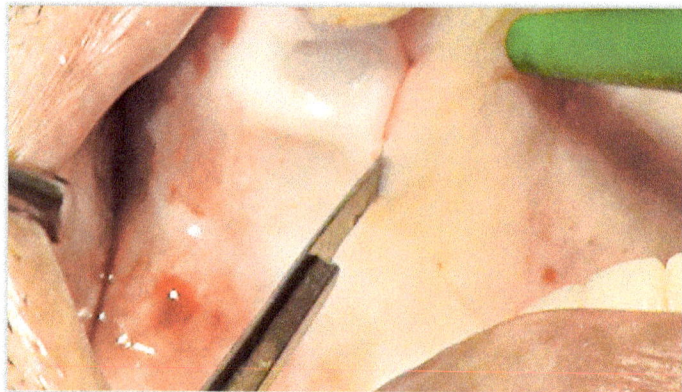

Fig. 6.4: Crestal incision placed slightly palatally.

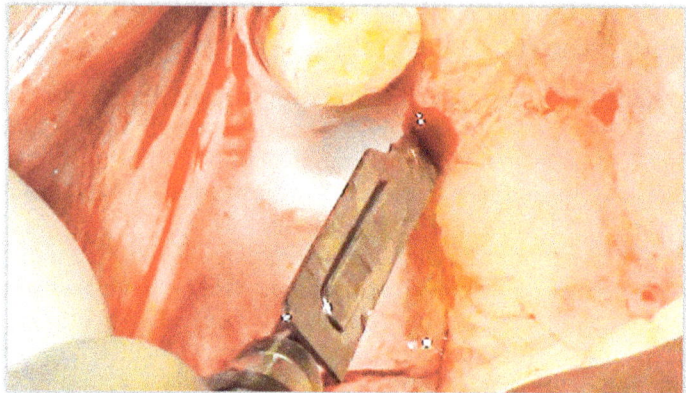

Fig. 6.5: Note distal releasing incision.

which may be close to the crest of the ridge in a severely atrophic maxilla. If uncontrolled bleeding occurs it may be stopped by a hemostat applied distal to the bleeding to constrict the artery. Pressure with a blunt instrument may also be applied over the palatine foramen. In most cases, pressure works the best.

A vertical release incision is made at least one tooth width away from the planned region of the bony window. The incision should not be extended beyond the vestibular sulcus. A distal vertical release incision may be made in case you wish to collect bone from the maxillary tuberosity (Fig. 6.5). The facial full thickness mucoperiosteal flap is reflected to expose completely the lateral wall of the maxilla and a part of the zygoma. The reflected labial tissue may be tied to the cheek mucosa with a stay suture (Fig. 6.6). All fibrous tissue should be removed from the lateral wall. At this stage, it would be a good idea to collect bone shavings from the lateral wall, zygoma and tuberosity area with bone scrapers or rongeurs for future use to be mixed with deproteinized bovine bone (Bio-Oss) (Fig. 6.7). It is also recommended that periosteal releasing incision be made at this stage for greater mobility of the facial flap and also to collect blood through a syringe with a wide bone needle (Fig. 6.8).

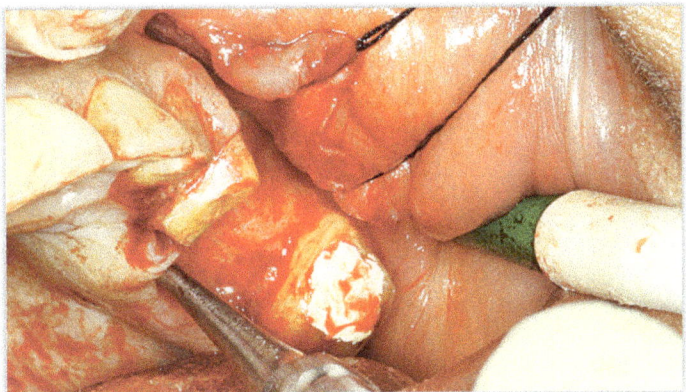

Fig. 6.6: Stay suture in place.

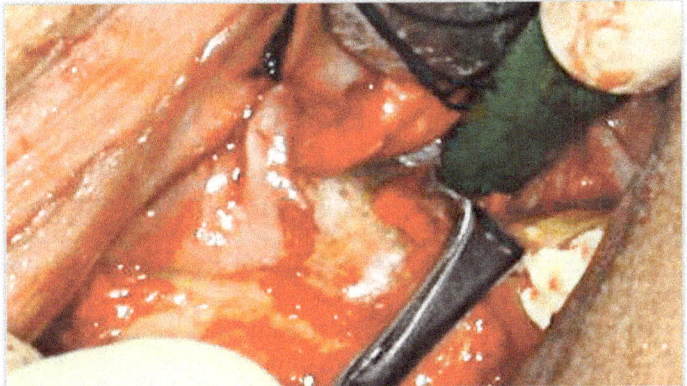

Fig. 6.7: Bone harvesting from the lateral wall of the sinus cavity.

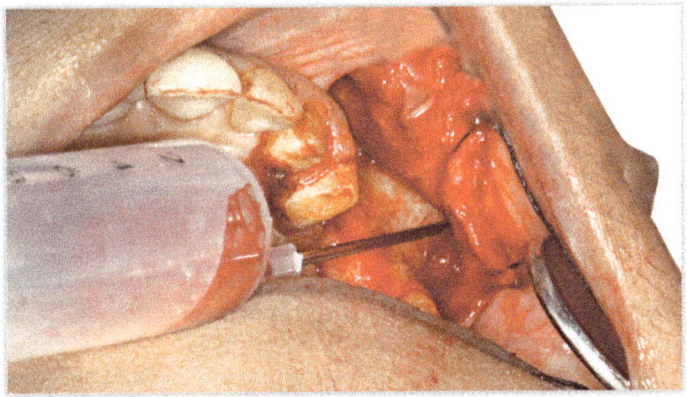

Fig. 6.8: Collecting blood with a large bore needle.

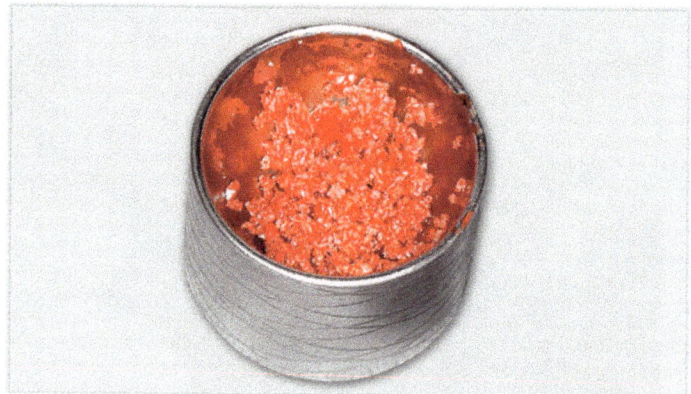

Fig. 6.9: Bio-Oss and autogenous bone chips mixed with fresh periosteal blood.

This collected blood is mixed with autogenous bone shavings and large particle size Bio-Oss to be used later as grafting material (Fig. 6.9).

ACCESS WINDOW TO THE SINUS CAVITY

The overall design of the lateral access window is determined by the radiographic examination which includes OPG as well as cone beam computed tomography (CBCT). The CBCT helps in determining the thickness of the lateral wall of the antrum, the distance of the antral floor from the crest of the ridge and the presence of septa on the floor and/or walls of the sinus.

The inferior margin of the window should be positioned 2-5 mm from the antral floor. If there is already a height of bone 5 mm from crest to the antral floor, you should mark the inferior margin 7 mm from the crest. If the inferior margin is made at or below the antral floor, removal of the bony window would be a problem possibly leading to a tear of the membrane. If the inferior margin is placed too high, more than 5 mm from the antral floor, dissection of the sinus membrane would be difficult as the operator would have to work without direct vision of the floor. The superior aspect of the access window should be about 6-8 mm from the inferior margin. The anterior vertical line should be about 3-4 mm distal to the anterior vertical wall of the antrum. It is better to err making a window over the antrum than into the bone surrounding the sinus. The distal vertical margin is about 10 mm from the anterior margin in the edentulous maxilla and should be in the region of the first molar which is within direct vision of the surgeon (Fig. 6.10). Although a larger access window offers advantage to the operator in terms of easier membrane elevation and sinus grafting because of better access, unnecessarily large window delays bone growth in the sinus because of the absence of the lateral bone sinus cavity.

The authors prefer starting the opening of the lateral access window with a no. 6 round carbide bur in a straight handpiece at a speed of 20,000 rpm. The bur is used in a light brushing motion and creates an outline of the window.

Sinus Grafting

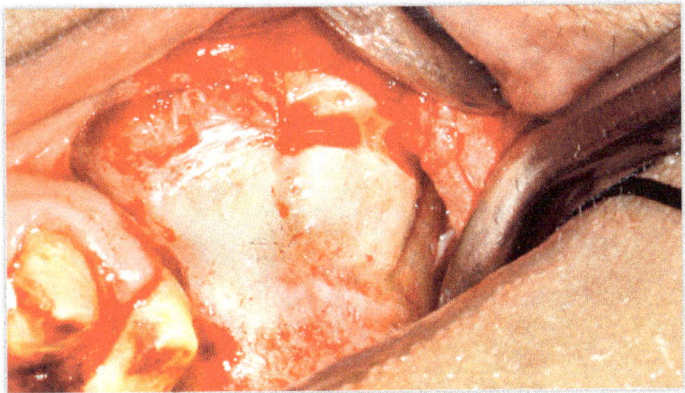

Fig. 6.10: Outline of the bony window with a no. 6 round carbide bur.

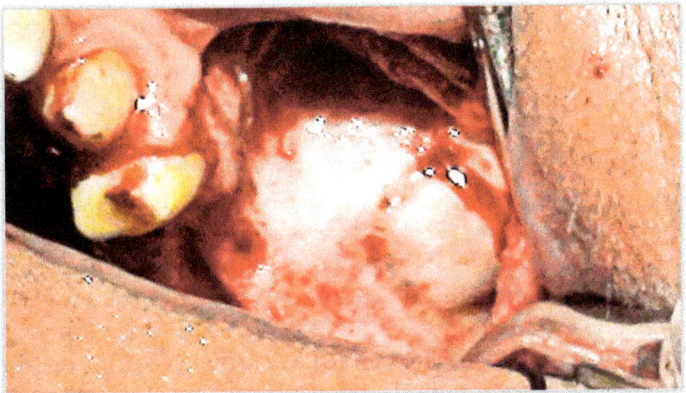

Fig. 6.11: Further deepening of the bony window with a no. 4 diamond showing the bluish membrane.

The bur is followed by a no. 4 round diamond which smoothens the bone between the grooves created by the carbide bur. Beginners may do the whole procedure using a no. 6 round diamond, since there are less chances of tearing the sinus membrane with a diamond as compared to a carbide bur. The corners of the access window should be rounded and not sharp because sharp corners can lead to perforation of the membrane during elevation by curettes at the corners. It can also cause tears in the membrane whilst removing the bony window. Once the lateral access window is delineated, the diamond bur continues in a paintbrush motion under saline irrigation till a bluish hue or hemorrhage is observed. The pneumatization of the sinus pushes the arteries of the membrane to surface just below the bone, therefore once the bluish hue or hemorrhage is observed, it is a sign that the membrane is reached (Fig. 6.11). Overpreparation should be avoided. To ensure that the bone has been prepared down to the membrane all the way round the oval osteotomy, it may be tapped gently and any movement may be observed. Alternatively, Piezosurgery using Sinus Surgery kit (Acteon India) is very predictable, with less chances of perforating the membrane. (Fig. 6.12)

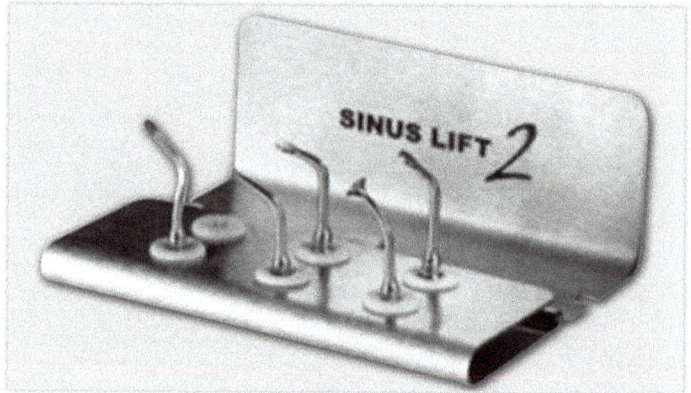

Fig. 6.12: Acteon sinus lift kit.

ELEVATION OF THE SINUS MEMBRANE

Elevation of the sinus membrane is done with the help of especially designed surgical curettes (Fig. 6.13). The authors prefer to separate the window from the membrane and remove it completely to be stored in saline for later replacement instead of inward fracturing (Fig. 6.14). Removing the bony window allows for better visualization and access (Fig. 6.15). Meticulous care should be taken to reflect the membrane superiorly without perforating. The lining of the sinus is first elevated from the floor and then from the medial wall of the sinus. It is also simultaneously extended towards the anterior and posterior walls. The curette is gently slid along the bone margin; this separates the membrane from the surrounding walls of the sinus (Fig. 6.16). Small motions of the instrument allow the margins to be lifted evenly. The tip of the instrument should be able to easily contact the bone, if not the opening may be widened with the diamond bur to gain better access. It is easier to gain direct vision and access to the posterior regions of the sinus cavity than the anterior region. Therefore, whenever the curette cannot stay with good contact against the bone and whenever access or visibility of the anterior region is poor one should not hesitate to extend the window anteriorly. The membrane should be elevated at at least 5 mm from the inferior edge of the window to gain adequate mobility. For the usual sinus window, the largest possible curette should be used to minimize the chances of perforation of the sinus. This is especially true as we enter deeper into the floor and the tension on the smaller curette increases.

Management of Perforation of the Sinus Membrane

The perforation of the Schneiderian (sinus) membrane has been reported to range from 10–30% of all lateral window sinus surgeries.[6] Perforations should be replaced with a collagen-based membrane like Bio-Gide (Geistlich Switzerland). It can be shaped into a dome and placed into the sinus to occlude the perforation and prevent the particulate graft from drifting (Fig. 6.17). It is however important to ensure that the sinus membrane has been completely lifted off the sinus floor so that the graft material does not rest on the epithelium but on the bare bony walls.

Sinus Grafting

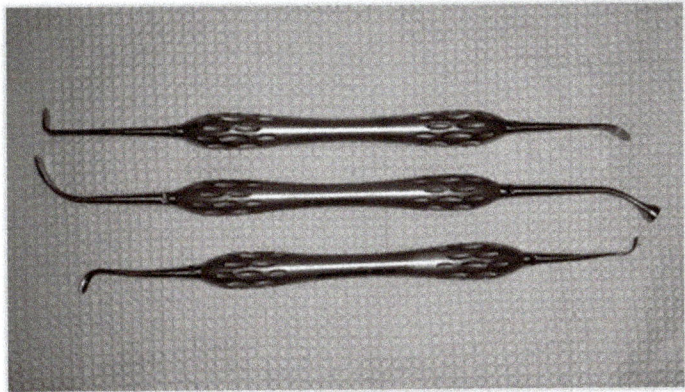

Fig. 6.13: Sinus membrane elevation curettes.

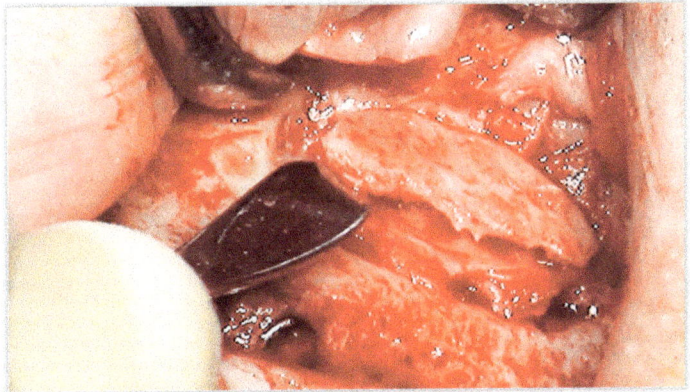

Fig. 6.14: Careful separation of the bony window from the sinus membrane with a sinus curette.

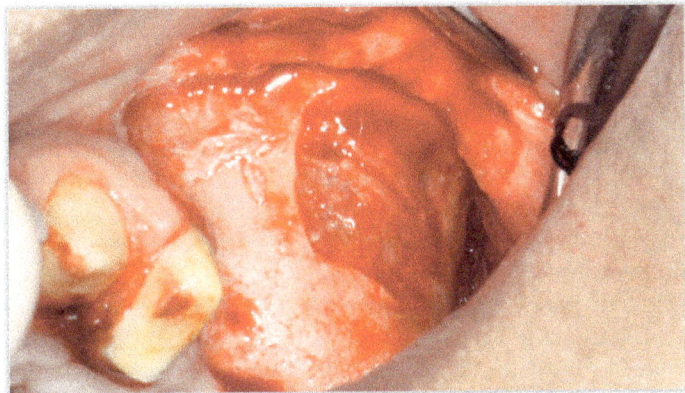

Fig. 6.15: Intact membrane after removal of bony window.

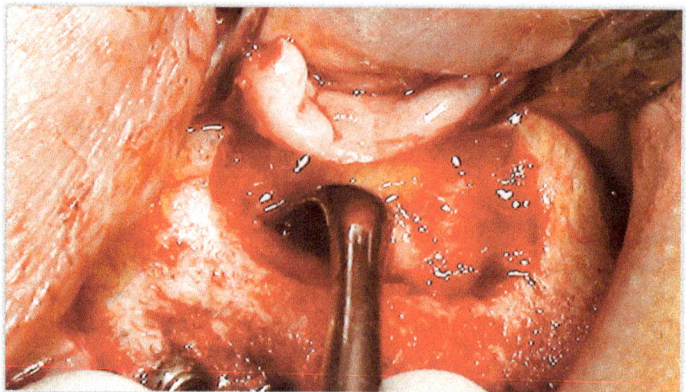

Fig. 6.16: Sliding the sinus curette between the membrane and the bone.

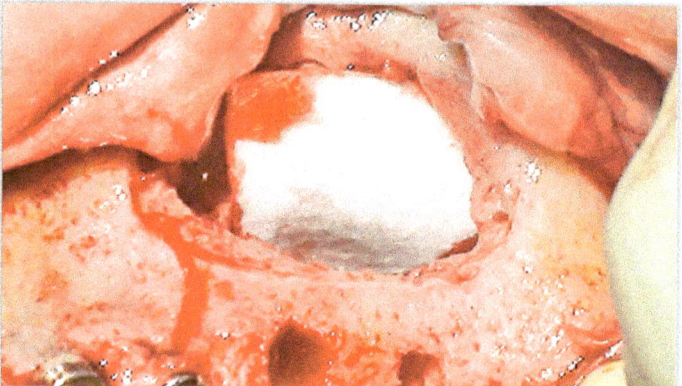

Fig. 6.17: Covering the perforation with a resorbable collagen membrane.

Sinus Graft Materials and Closure of the Lateral Access Window

It is reported in the literature that the mere lifting of the sinus membrane and tenting it by the simultaneous placement of implants, is sufficient for bone to grow inside the sinus cavity. However, the authors adopt a more reliable and time tested method of keeping the sinus membrane raised by grafting the sinus cavity with a slowly resorbing space maintaining biomaterial (Fig. 6.18) and covering the same with the original bony window (Fig. 6.19). In cases where the window does not approximate well to the walls of the access window, it is preferable to cover the same with a noncross-linked resorbable collagen membrane like Bio-Gide (Fig. 6.20). A large variety of bone substitute materials are available including allogenic, xenogenic and synthetic bone graft materials. One of the most documented is a bovine bone consisting of deproteinized

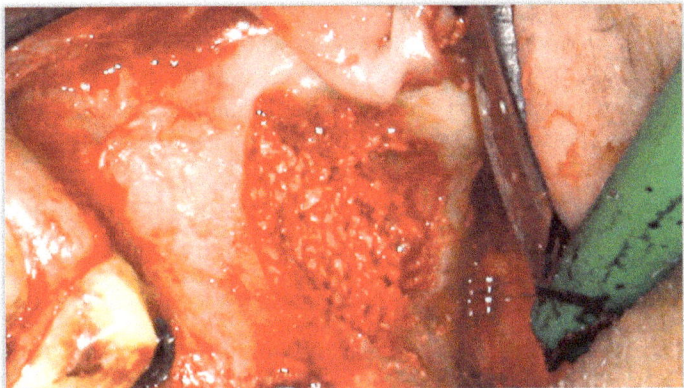

Fig. 6.18: Grafting the sinus cavity and keeping the membrane elevated.

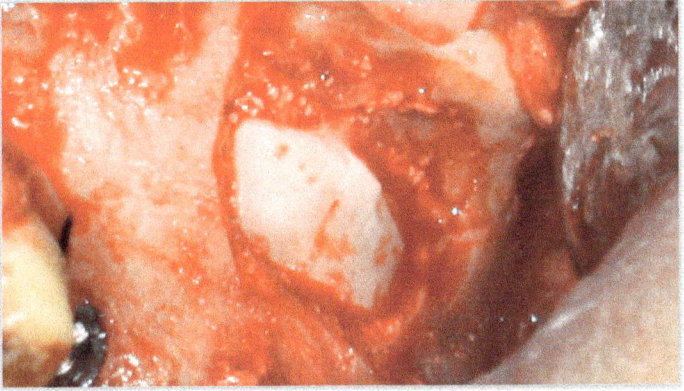

Fig. 6.19: Replacing the lateral bony window.

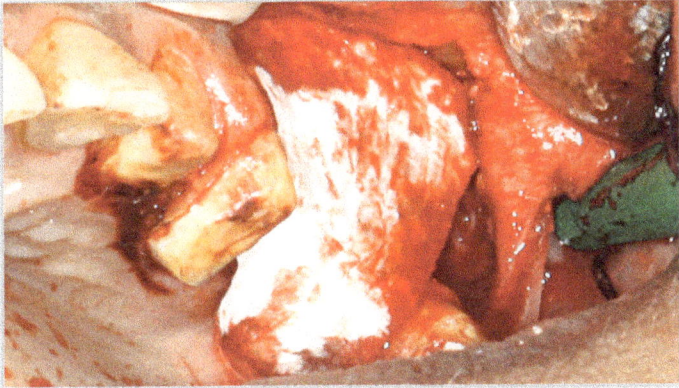

Fig. 6.20: Covering the replaced bony window with a collagen membrane.

bovine bone mineral (Bio-Oss). The material has been shown to integrate well with bone and resorbs very slowly with time. Since the material does not have any bone inductive potential, the authors usually mix it with bone scrapings locally harvested from the lateral wall of the maxilla and tuberosity (see Fig. 6.7). The material can also be used on its own but then the period of bone formation will be longer (at least 6 months).

COMPLICATIONS

Infection of the Grafted Sinus Cavity

Infection of the grafted sinus cavity fortunately is not common, especially if the patient is prescribed pre- and postoperative antibiotics for a period of 7 days. The drug of choice is Amoxicillin with Clavulanic Acid 625 mg, twice a day (Tresmox CV, Abbott India) because of its documented activity against aerobes and anaerobes. Patients allergic to Penicillin can be safely prescribed Clindamycin 300 mg (Dalacin-C Pfizer, India) three times a day. In few patients after the initial healing period, they may experience an infection of the grafted sinus which can be controlled and resolved by again prescribing the same antibiotic three times a day for a period of 7 days. In the experience of the authors, they have had to do, in only one case a re-entry and remove the entire grafted material. However, the case was a diabetic and had not followed the antibiotic protocol properly.

Incision Line Opening

Incision line opening may be a problem especially when the wound is closed under tension with not adequate periosteal releasing incision (Fig. 6.21). However, this complication if the patient is on chlorhexidine rinses (Periogard, Colgate, India), this opening heals by secondary intention by the formation of granulation tissue (Fig. 6.22).

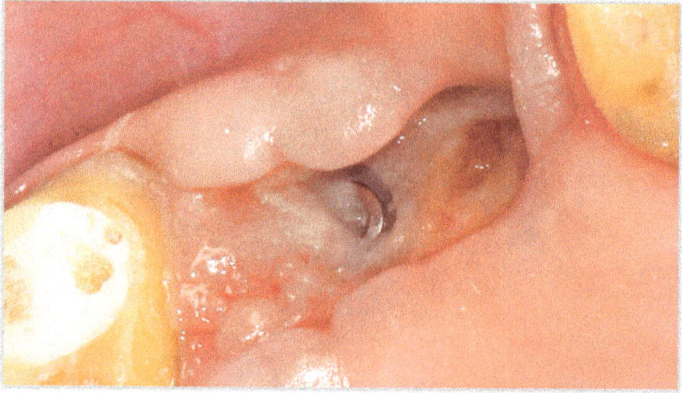

Fig. 6.21: Incision line opening and part exposure of implant after a period of 7 days.

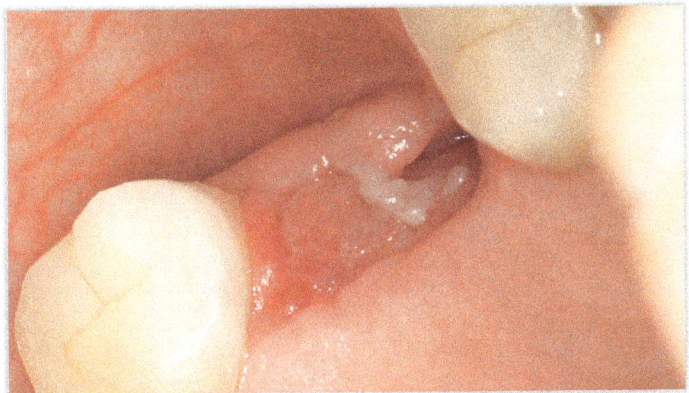

Fig. 6.22: Healing by secondary intention, 18 days after surgery.

CASE REPORT

Male patient aged 70 years has lost all his posterior teeth in the upper jaw and now requests to be rehabilitated with fixed prosthesis.

Diagnosis and Treatment planning

On examination, it is noticed that his remaining six natural teeth are not in good health and will also require treatment (Fig. 6.23). Panoramic X-ray shows that there is very little bone height posterior to the canine to place implants (Fig. 6.24). The patient was explained that he would require bilateral sinus grafting using a lateral window approach and later implant placement in a staged procedure. It was also explained that the total treatment time would be about one year. The patient agreed to the above treatment line.

Surgical Procedures

Since the available bone from the crest of the ridge to the floor of the sinus was only 2-3 mm, it was decided to do a staged approach with grafting, waiting for 6-8 months for bone to grow in the grafted sinus and then do another surgery for placement of the implants. Accordingly, on the left side, lateral window sinus graft surgery was undertaken on 21st January, 2009 (Figs. 6.25 to 6.34). On opening of the lateral window, it was observed that there was clearly a bony septa incompletely separating the sinus cavity into an anterior and posterior compartment (Fig. 6.31). Therefore, utmost care was taken to very carefully separate and lift the membrane. Although septa in the sinus are difficult to manage during grafting they are also advantageous because they act as an additional bony wall for blood vessels to grow into the graft and form bone. Especially designed sinus curettes were used to carefully lift the membrane from the floor of the sinus taking great care to see that the curette always remained in contact with the floor of the sinus. This is a very delicate

82 Clinical Guide to Oral Implantology: Step by Step Procedures

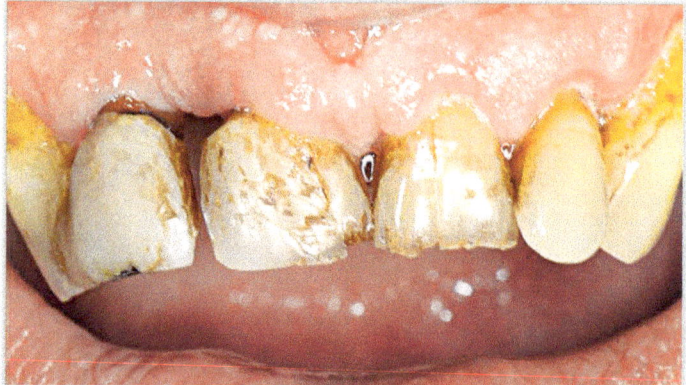

Fig. 6.23: Preoperative intraoral view.

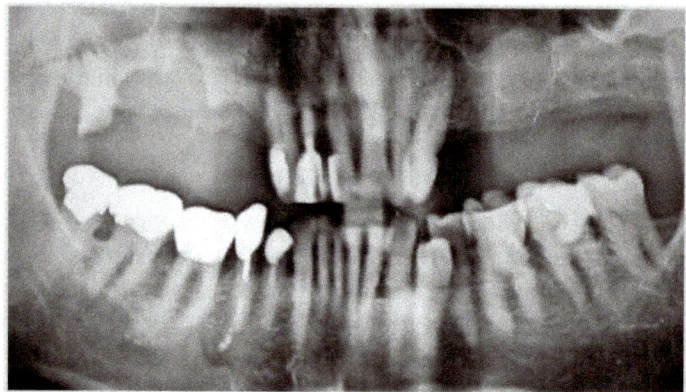

Fig. 6.24: Preoperative OPG.

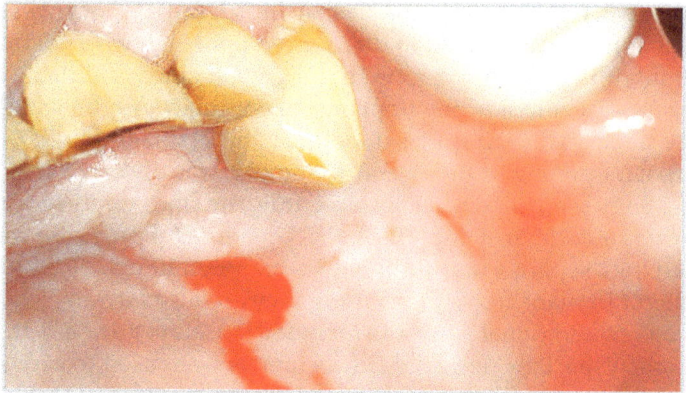

Fig. 6.25: Preoperative intraoral view of left side.

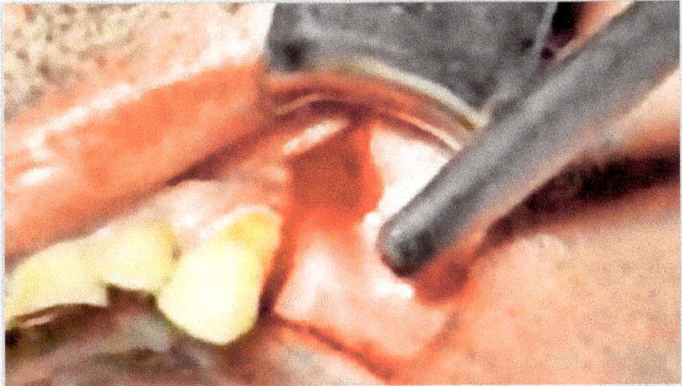

Fig. 6.26: Incision.

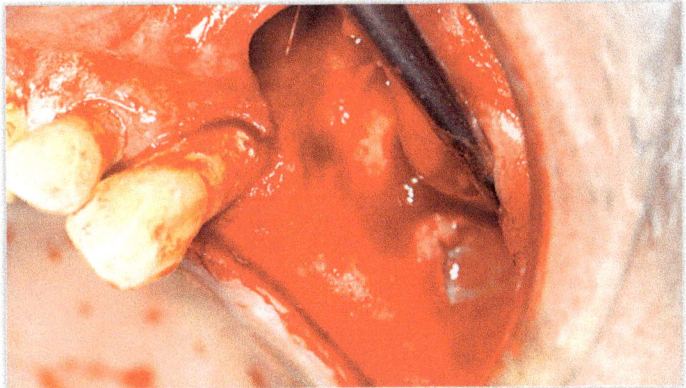

Fig. 6.27: Reflected view of surgical site.

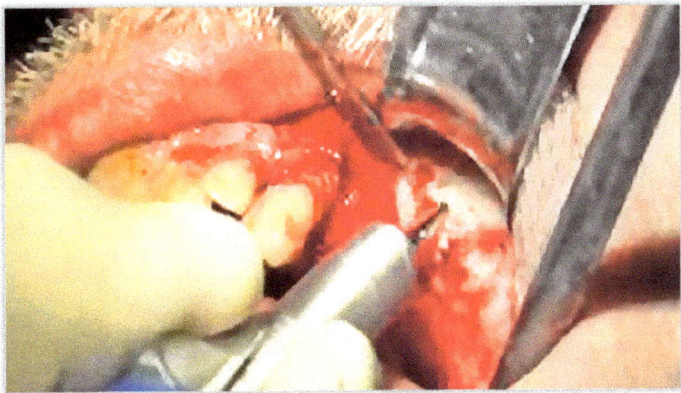

Fig. 6.28: Drilling of window outline.

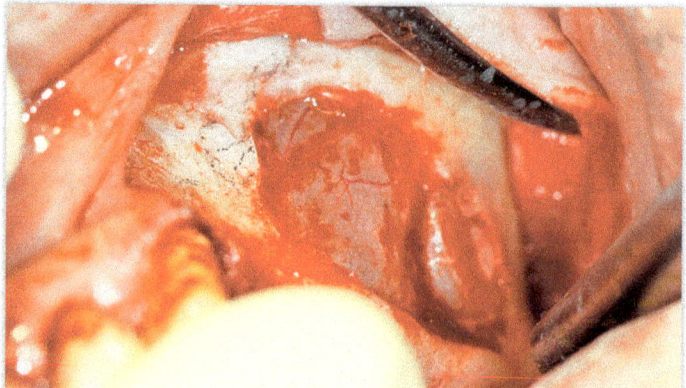

Fig. 6.29: View after removal of bony window.

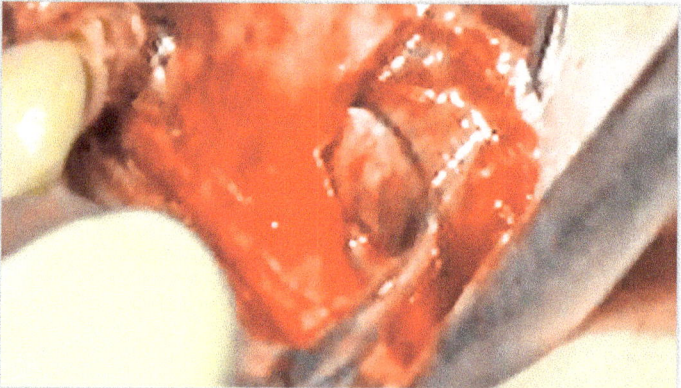

Fig. 6.30: Membrane elevation.

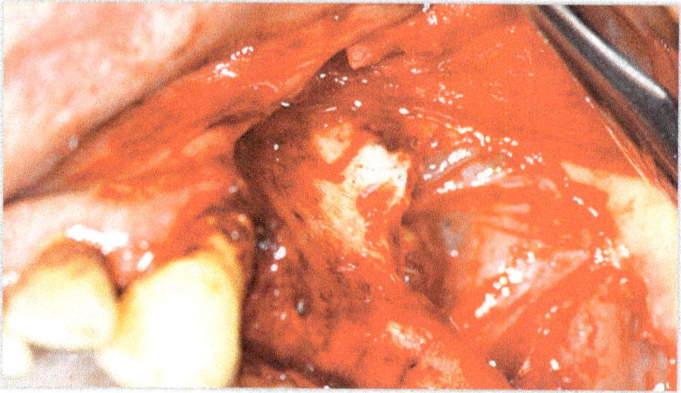

Fig. 6.31: Elevated membrane also showing incomplete bony septa.

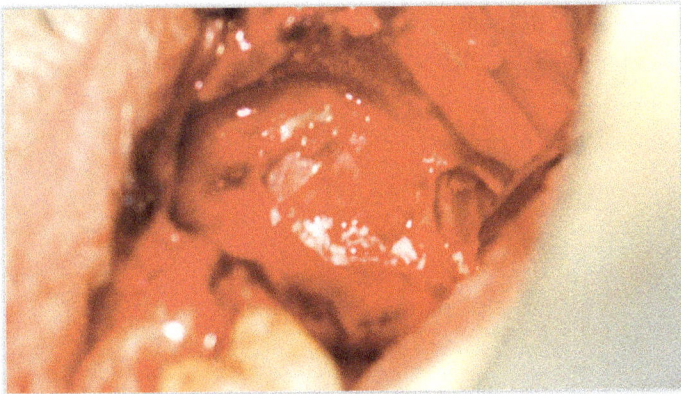

Fig. 6.32: Bone grafting with Bio-Oss.

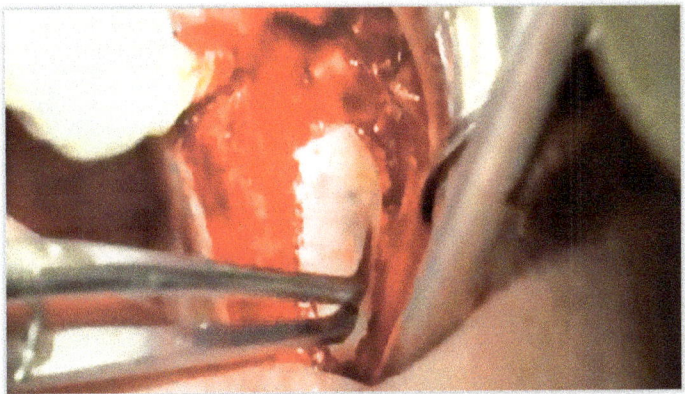

Fig. 6.33: Placing back the bony window.

procedure and under no circumstances should one be in a hurry to accomplish the same. The authors prefer to lift off the bony window and keep it in saline for later replacement, in preference to the method of fracturing the bony window and lifting the same along with the membrane. Since the window is replaced back, the authors believe that at times there is no need to cover the grafted lateral wall with a membrane before closure of the wound. The nonuse of a membrane also makes this technique economical (Fig. 6.33).

After waiting for a period of one month for recovery from the first surgery, a similar lateral wall sinus grafting was done on the right side on 23.2.2009 (Figs. 6.35 and 6.36)

Looking at the advanced age of the patient and the large windows that had to be prepared it was decided to wait for 8 months for bone to form in the grafted sites before placement of implants. (Fig. 6.37) shows the OPG taken 8 months after the sinus grafting. During this period, the anterior teeth were rehabilitated (Fig. 6.38).

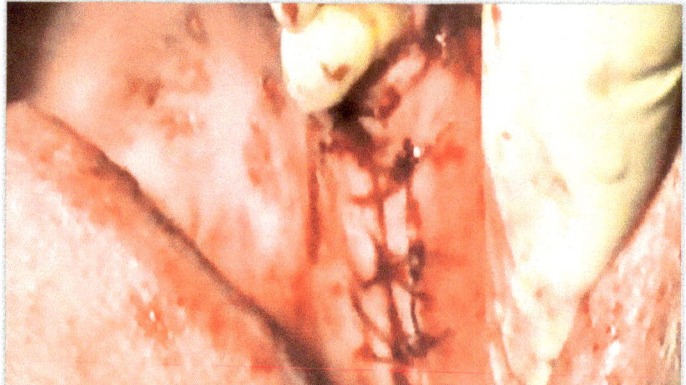

Fig. 6.34: Placing back the flap and suturing.

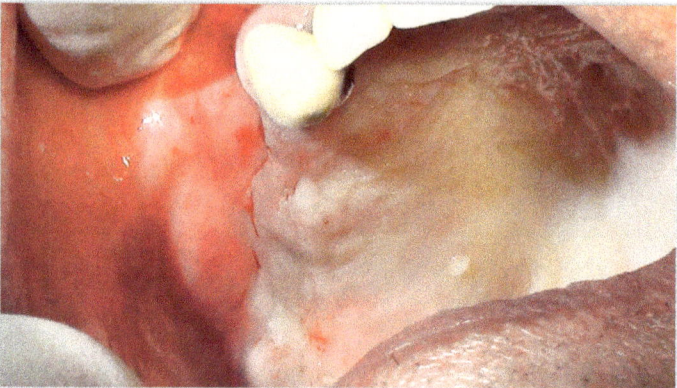

Fig. 6.35: Preoperative view of right side.

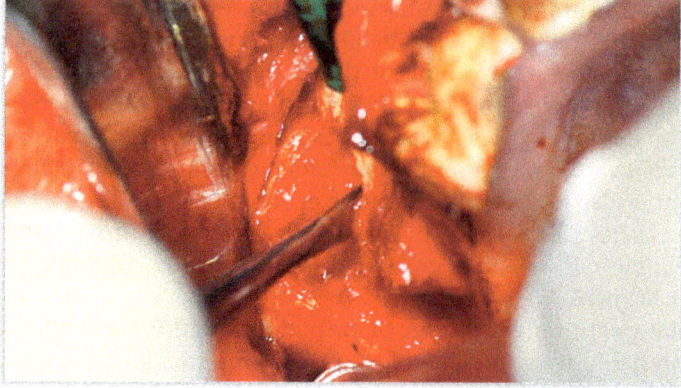

Fig. 6.36: Elevation of the membrane on the right side.

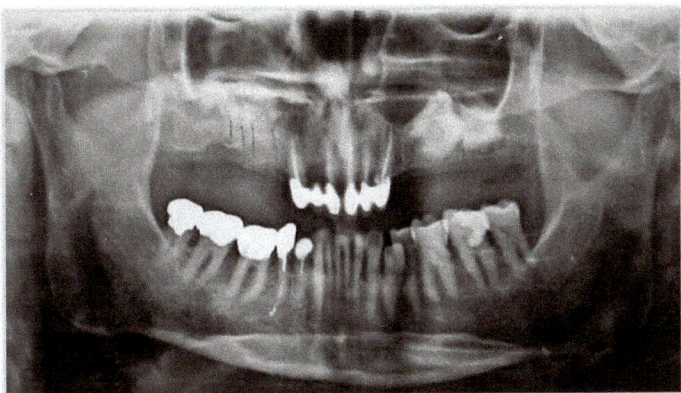

Fig. 6.37: OPG after grafting.

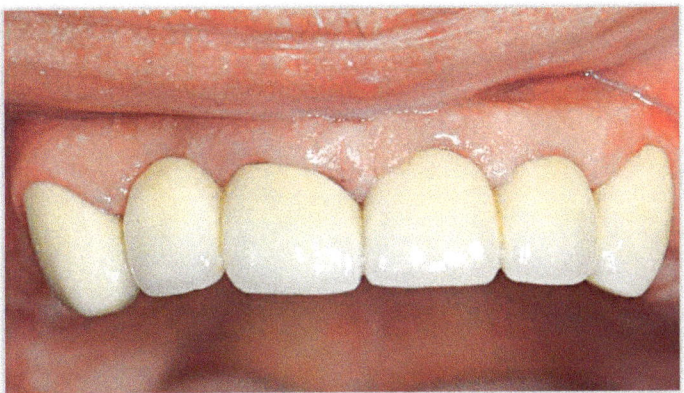

Fig. 6.38: Waiting for bone to grow in sinus cavity and patient was rehabilitated with anterior aesthetic fixed prosthesis.

Implant surgery consisted of 3 implants placed on the left side in the region of the first premolar, second premolar and first molar (Figs. 6.39 to 6.41). A vacuum formed surgical stent on a model prepared by duplicating a wax up of the final prosthesis was used as a guide. Subsequently implants were placed on the right side (Figs. 6.42 to 6.44).

It was decided to do one stage surgical placement of implants keeping the implants non-submerged thus avoiding second stage surgery. The implants selected were ANKYLOS Implants (Dentsply Sirona Implants, Germany). The progressive thread design of the "ANKYLOS" tapered screw ensures good primary stability even in poor quality bone which was to be expected in the grafted sinuses. Implant to Bone Contact (BIC) was further optimized by using Ankylos system which has a grit blasted and thermally acid etched surface (Plus Surface, Dentsply Sirona Implants). The implant in the upper right first molar was left submerged because it did not exhibit very good stability.

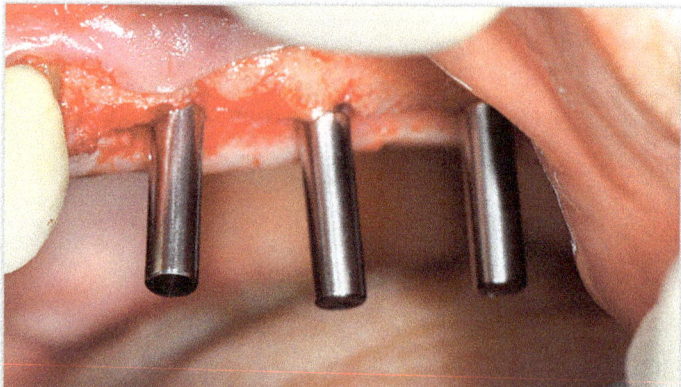

Fig. 6.39: Paralleling pins placed.

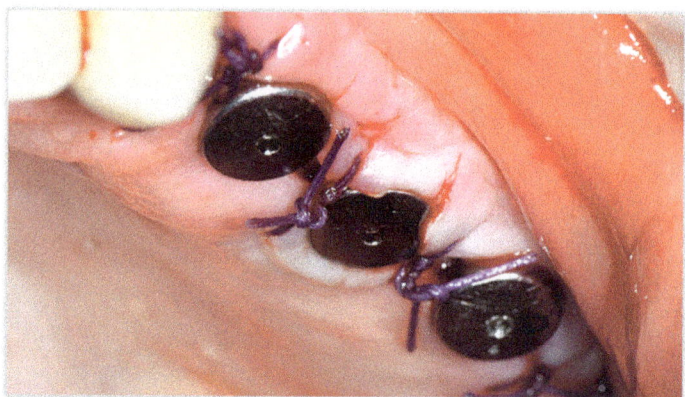

Fig. 6.40: Cover screws removed and sulcus formers placed thus avoiding second stage surgery.

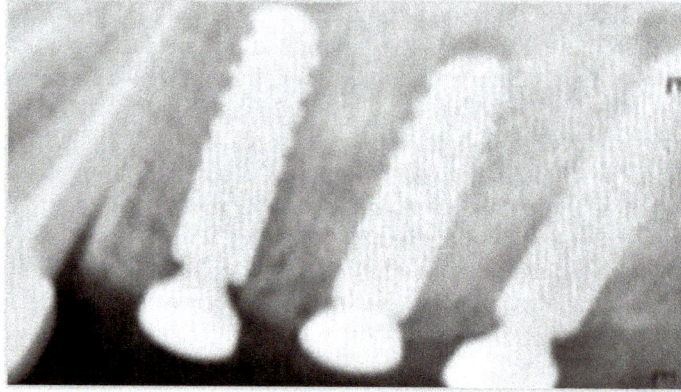

Fig. 6.41: Radiographic view after implant placement on left side.

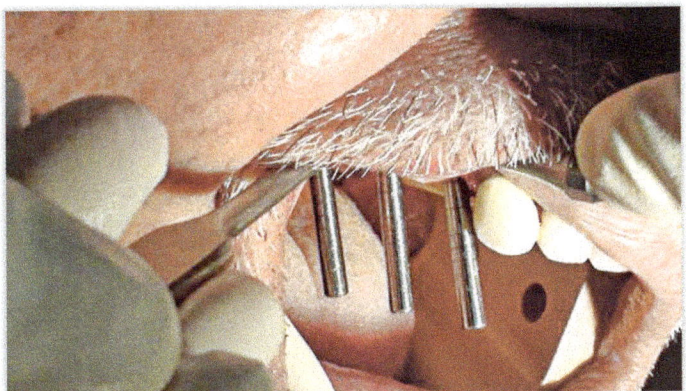

Fig. 6.42: Paralleling pins in place on right side.

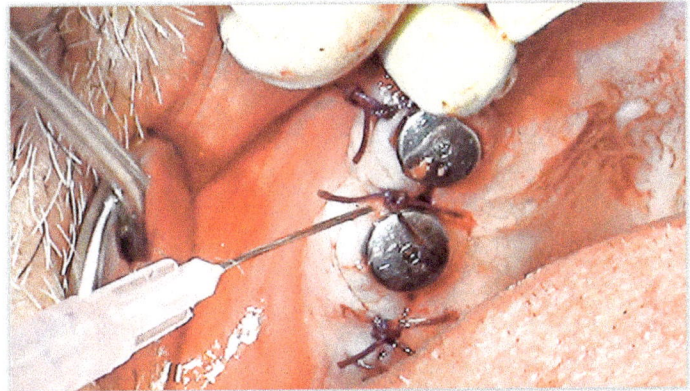

Fig. 6.43: Implants placed on right side after 8 months.

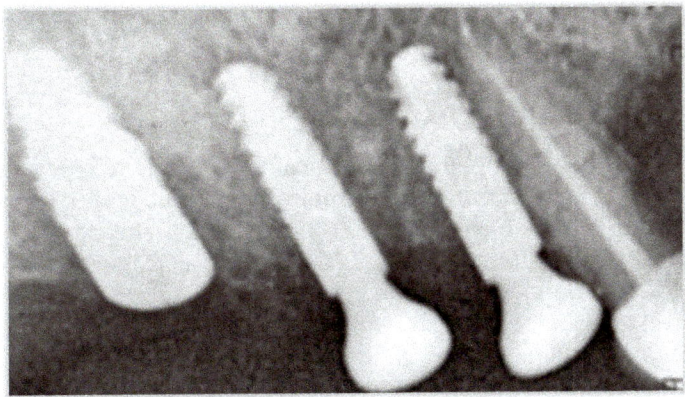

Fig. 6.44: Radiographic view of implants on right side.
Note: Implant placed in first molar region is submerged.

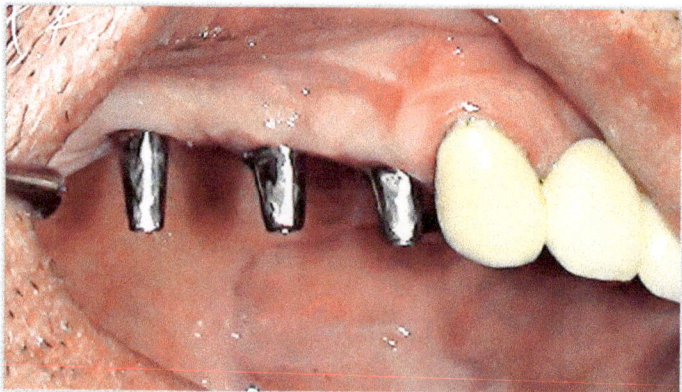

Fig. 6.45: Abutments in place on right side.

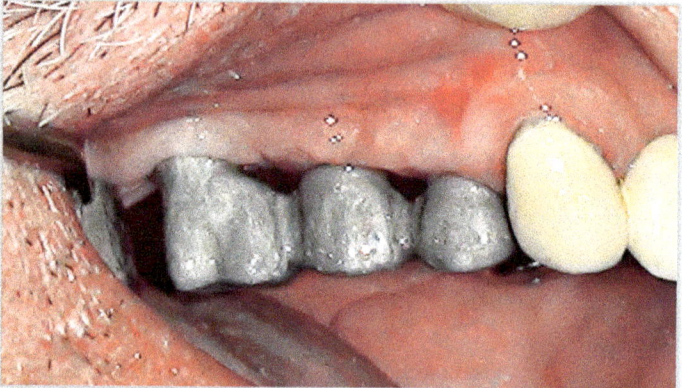

Fig. 6.46: Metal try-in on right side.

After a period of 4 months, the prosthetic part of the rehabilitation was commenced (Figs. 6.45 to 6.55).

Maintenance of Sinus Surgery Patients

The risk of suture line opening and exposure of the grafted area is one of the most annoying and serious complication after sinus graft surgery. Besides systemic antibiotics local antibacterial agents like chlorhexidine must be prescribed to the patient. Periogard (Colgate India) is the most documented chlorhexidine mouth wash which has been shown to prevent infection of the graft even after incision line opening. It is available in 0.12% Chlorhexidine in alcohol base. Patients are told to gargle with Periogard at least twice a day keeping the mouthwash in the mouth for 30 seconds. It may be increased to 3 times a day in case of incision line opening as had occurred in the present case (Figs. 6.21 and 6.22)

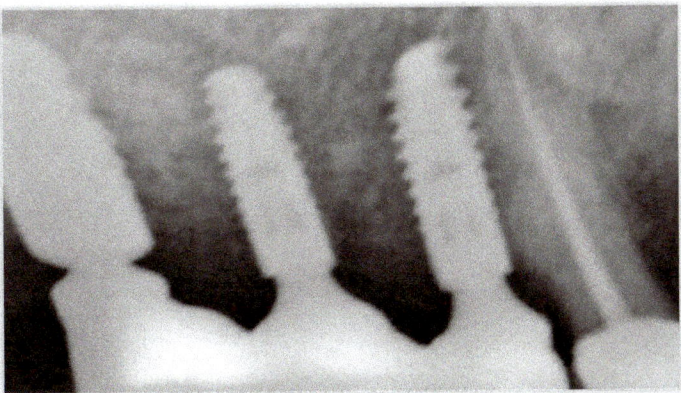

Fig. 6.47: Radiographic view of metal try-in. *Note:* Excellent marginal fit.

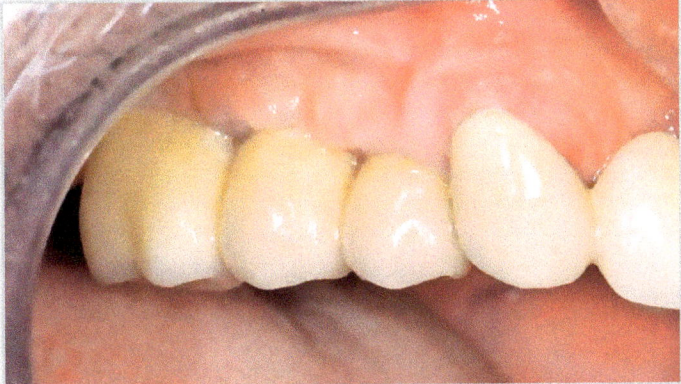

Fig. 6.48: Final porcelain-fused-to-metal (PFM) crowns splinted on right side.

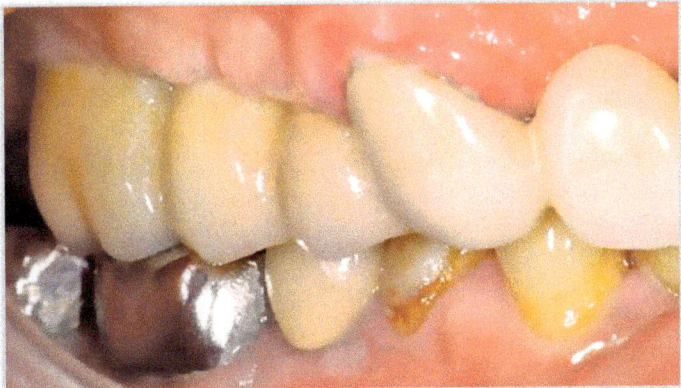

Fig. 6.49: View in occlusion on right side.

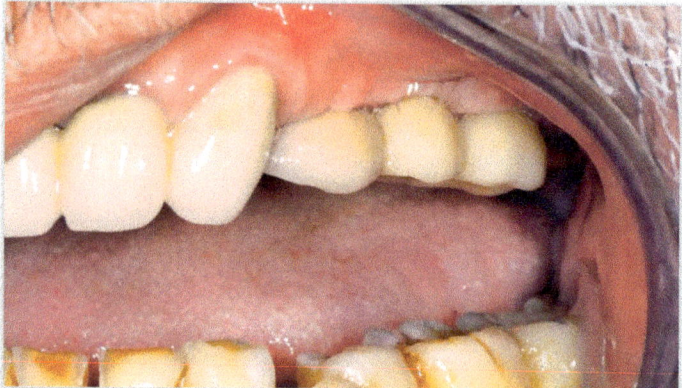

Fig. 6.50: Final porcelain-fused-to-metal (PFM) splinted crowns on left side.

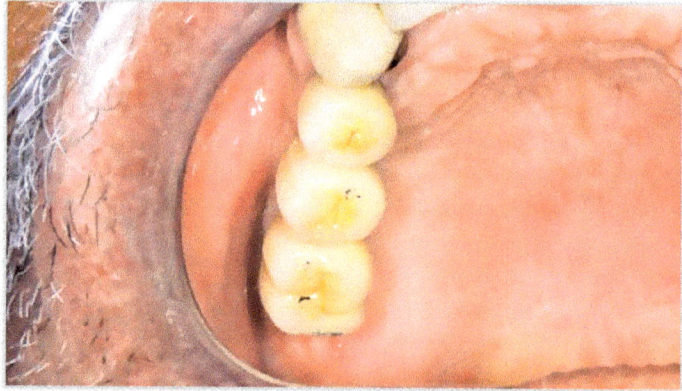

Fig. 6.51: Intraoral occlusal view, note that with the ankylos system. It is possible to duplicate the natural anatomy of lost teeth without reducing their size.

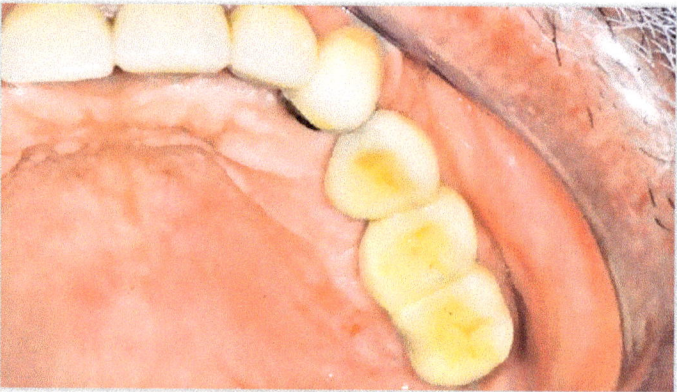

Fig. 6.52: Intraoral occlusal view, left side.

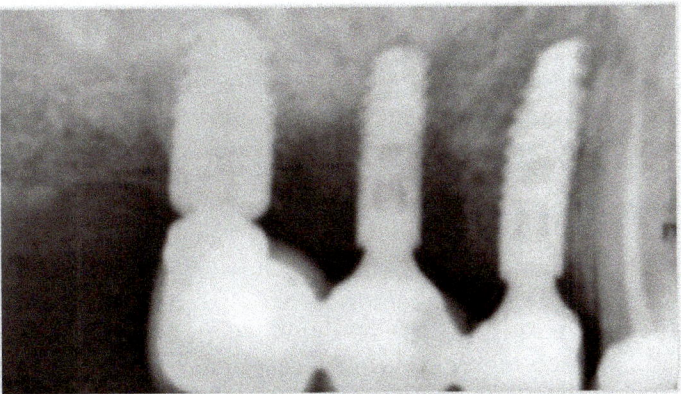

Fig. 6.53: Radiograph showing excellent marginal fit of cemented porcelain-fused-to-metal (PFM) splinted crowns on right side.

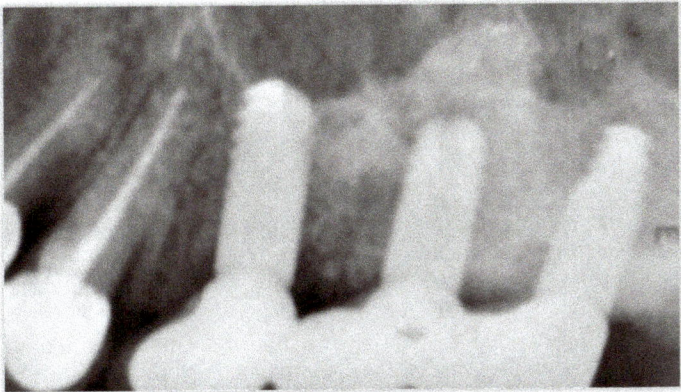

Fig. 6.54: Radiograph showing excellent marginal fit of cemented porcelain-fused-to-metal (PFM) splinted crowns on the left side.

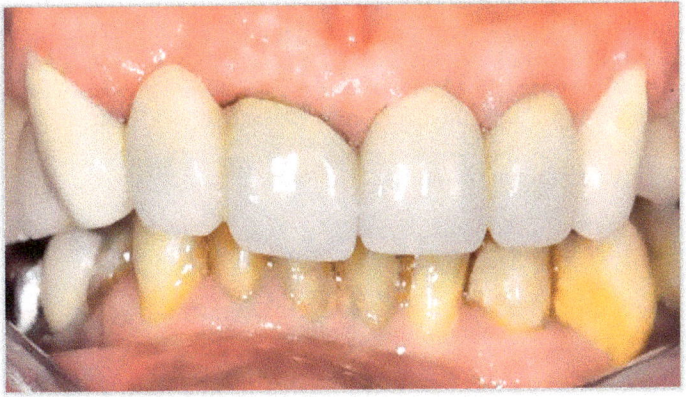

Fig. 6.55: Postoperative intraoral view.

It is also important to prescribe an ultra soft toothbrush (Colgate Slim Soft) and an antibacterial fluoride tooth paste containing Triclosan and the polymer Gantrez which give it long lasting effect (Colgate Total Toothpaste). It is the authors opinion that the present case of incision line opening and subsequent resolution of the lesion was due to aggressive local measures outlined earlier.

DISCUSSION

There are two options for rehabilitation of missing upper posterior teeth. The first and the simplest is by a removable cast partial denture. However, most patients are unable to function well with the same especially when the ridges are resorbed, as was the situation in this case report. Incidentally, a removable cast partial denture was fabricated for this patient whilst waiting for healing after sinus grafting but was not accepted by the patient. The second option and more difficult one is to do sinus grafting in a one stage procedure with simultaneous implant placement (if enough bone is present for primary stability of the implants). This is the procedure the authors prefer in most case even if 3-4 mm of bone is available, since it saves time and the number of surgeries are reduced. However, in this particular case where there was poor quality and quantity of bone available it was decided to do a staged procedure. Therefore, the total rehabilitation time took about 1 year and 3 months.

REFERENCES

1. Tatum OH. Maxillary Sinus Grafting for End osseous Implants. Presented at the Annual meeting at the Alabama Implant Study Group, April, 1977, Birmingham, AL.
2. Boyne PJ, James RA. Grafting of the maxillary sinus floor with autogenous marrow and bone. J Oral Surg. 1980;38:613-6.
3. Lundgren S, Andersson S, Gualini F, et al. Bone reformation with sinus membrane elevation: A new surgical technique for maxillary sinus floor augmentation. Clin Implant Dent Relat Res. 2004;6: 165-73.
4. Palma VC, Magro-Filho O, de Oliveira JA, et al. Bone reformation and implant integration following maxillary sinus membrane elevation: An experimental study in primates . Clin Oral Implants Res. 2006;8:11-24.
5. Nedir R, Bischof M, Vazquez L, et al. Osteotome sinus floor elevation without grafting material: A 1- year prospective pilot study with ITI Implants. Clin Oral Implants Res. 2006;17:679-86.
6. Jensen OT, Leonard BS, Block MS, et al. Report of the sinus consensus conference of 1996, Int J Oral Maxillofac Implants. 1998;13(suppl):11-30.

Chapter 7

Crestal Sinus Floor Elevation

The atrophic maxilla especially in the posterior region due to the presence of the maxillary sinus have very little height of bone present to place dental implants. The sinus bony cavity is lined by a specialized type of periosteum which is rather delicate and is lined by ciliated, columnar epithelial cells, which continuously helps in removing mucous and other foreign material from the sinus through the ostium situated in the middle meatus of the nasal cavity. Air flows into and out of the maxillary sinus during inspiration and expiration respectively. The increase in size of the sinus cavity (pneumatization) occurs continuously throughout life and increases with age and after tooth loss.[1]

Various techniques to augment bone by lifting the sinus membrane and growing bone in the air-filled cavity in order to place implants have been introduced. They include the lateral window technique first published by Boyne and James in 1980.[2]

In 1994, Summers introduced the crestal approach for sinus grafting by the use of especially designed osteotomes to break the sinus floor by bone compaction at the same time improve the quality of bone by lateral condensation.[3] Even though the lateral window technique has been proven to be a reliable technique for sinus augmentation, this technique results in considerable postoperative pain, swelling, discomfort and possibility of infection.[4] Summers technique of crestal sinus floor elevation depends on bone compaction to elevate the sinus membrane through the use of osteotomes which has some limitations such as possible sinus membrane perforation from compaction of the bone. In addition malleting by osteotomes can lead to post-operative vertigo due to trauma to the inner ear.[5] Also the osteotome-mediated sinus floor elevation (OMSFE) has lower success rates when residual bone height is less than 4 mm.[6] Breaking the sinus floor using OMSFE in the steep anterior wall of the sinus cavity and septum area may be difficult because of dense bone.

To combine the advantages of piezoelectric surgery to break the sinus floor first introduced by Vercellotti in 2000[7] with internal irrigation to raise the sinus membrane evenly both from medially and laterally, Sohn et al. popularized the hydrodynamic piezoelectric internal sinus floor elevation (HPISE).[8]

The authors prefer to use the Intra Lift Kit developed by Acteon (France) to break the sinus floor and enlarge the osteotomy sequentially (Fig. 7.1).

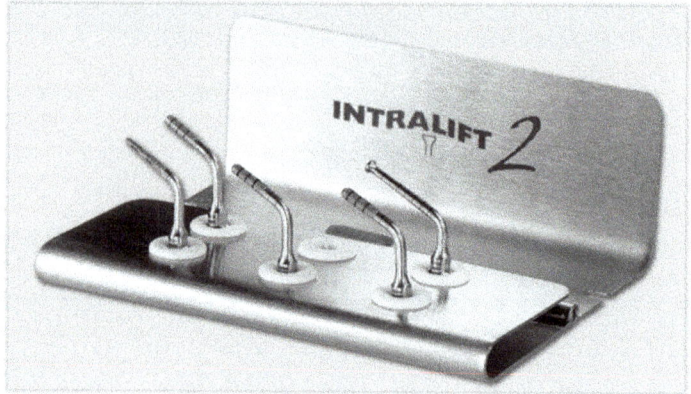

Fig. 7.1: Intralift kit (Acteon).

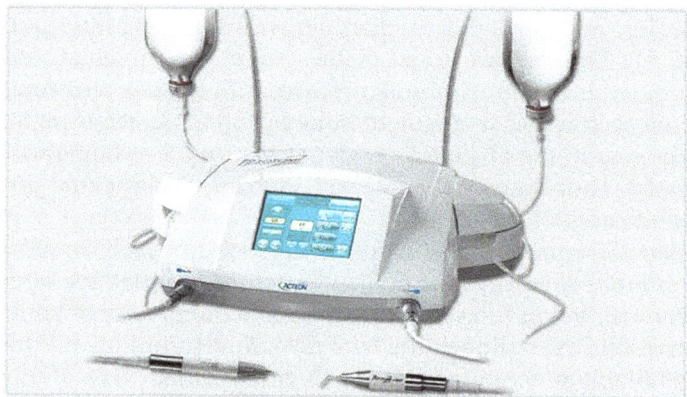

Fig. 7.2: Piezotome 2 (Acteon).

If the height of the bone from the crest to the sinus floor is less than 4 mm, then there is no need to use the surgical drill and you can start with using piezoelectric microvibrations from TKW1, TKW2, TKW3, TKW4 intra lift tips. The tips have to be used with gentle pressure and with maximum irrigation setting with the Piezotome 2 (Acteon, France) (Fig. 7.2). Gentle pressure and maximum irrigation is required in order to prevent overheating of the bone which would result in necrosis and loss of bone. Since no rotary drills are used to break the sinus floor nor osteotomes but instead microvibration created through piezoelectric, there are minimal chances of perforating the sinus membrane. Subsequently bone compaction is not used to elevate the sinus membrane, instead the internal irrigation from the TKW5 is used to elevate the sinus membrane evenly before introduction of any grafting material (Fig. 7.3).

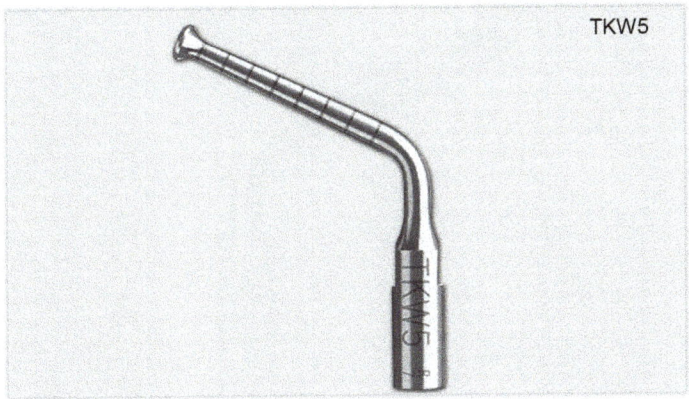

Fig. 7.3: Insert with internal irrigation to elevate the membrane.

SURGICAL TECHNIQUE

After local anesthesia using lignocaine 2% with 1:80000 adrenaline in the surgical site a full thickness mucoperiosteal flap is elevated to expose the alveolar ridge. Flapless surgery may also be performed when the width of the alveolar ridge is more than 7 mm. Usually, the TKW2 tip with a diameter of 2.1 mm is used to break the sinus floor. Further enlargement is done with the TKW3 and TKW4 tips. The TKW4 tip has the final diameter of 2.8 mm (Fig. 7.4). Next the elevation of the sinus membrane is done with the TKW5 which has internal irrigation. To prevent perforation of the sinus membrane, the water pressure can be reduced to 70 mm and elevation should be done for about 10 sec. This procedure should be repeated once again for even elevation of the sinus membrane both laterally and mesially. The integrity of the membrane can be confirmed with the Valsalva's maneuver or direct visualization. The backflow of saline from the sinus cavity during application of hydrolytic pressure also confirms the integrity of the sinus membrane. After this procedure when the height of the bone is less the surgeon can observe the up and down movement of the sinus membrane on asking the patient to inhale and exhale.

The bone graft material preferred by the authors is a bovine bone mineral (Bio-Oss, Geistlich), which is a well-documented osteoconductive biosubstitute. It can be used in particulate form mixed with saline or still better mixed with autologous fibrin glue which makes it sticky and prevents its migration. If autologous fibrin glue is not available, it is better to use Bio-Oss Collagen (Geistlich) which is 90% Bio-Oss and 10 % collagen. Bio-Oss collagen like sticky bone does not migrate and thus even if the membrane is ruptured the material will not migrate and block the ostium. Bone compaction is attained by using the ultrasonic vibration of the piezoelectric device by using the TKW5 with gentle water irrigation of 70 mm. This negates the need to use physical pressure to pack the bone graft, thereby reducing the possibility of membrane perforation. If you are using an implant of upto 4.5 mm in diameter, then the TKW4 insert is the last instrument to make the osteotomy prior to implant placement. When a wider implant is to be placed say a 5.5 mm, intermittent

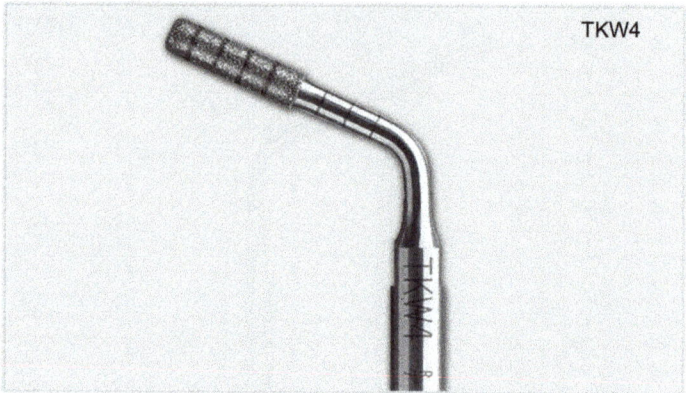

Fig. 7.4: The final insert of diameter 2.8 mm

drilling will be required to accommodate the wider diameter implant. However, always the osteotomy should be undersized by one drill in order to achieve adequate primary stability of the implant.

CASE 1

A 44-year-old male patient who wanted an implant supported fixed prosthesis replacing his lost teeth nos 24 and 25. Preoperative plain intraoral radiographs showed residual bone height of about 7 mm in the 24 region and about 5 mm in the 25 region.

The width of the bone on mapping was only about 5.5 mm in the 24 region and about 6 mm in the 25 region. A buccal concavity was also observed in the region between 24 and 25 (Fig. 7.5). It was therefore decided not to do flapless. A mucoperiosteal flap, was reflected without any vertical incision (Fig. 7.6). In site 24, normal osteotomy with Ankylos system of Dentsply Sirona Implants was done to a height of about 6 mm, after which the Acteon intralift inserts were used to break the sinus floor (Fig. 7.7). In site 25 region, the osteotomy was done completely with the Intralift kit starting with TKW1 up to a depth of about 4 mm. The floor of the sinus was the broken with the TKW2. The osteotomy was then enlarged with the TKW3 and TKW4. Finally, the TKW5 with irrigation was used to elevate the sinus membrane in both 24 and 25 osteotomies. The Valsalva's maneuver confirmed that the membrane was not ruptured. Bio-Oss small particle with amalgam carrier was subsequently compacted under the raised membrane with the help of the ultrasonic energy and irrigation from the TKW5 (Fig. 7.8). Two Ankylos implants (Dentsply Sirona) 3.5 × 9.5 mm were placed simultaneously with good primary stability because of the undersizing of the osteotomies (Fig. 7.9). Intraoral plain radiographs taken immediately after placement shows that in site 25 about five threads of the implant are inside the sinus cavity. Sulcus formers were placed and non-submerged healing for 6 months was allowed for growth of bone in the sinus cavity. After 6 months at the time of impression making excellent bone growth was observed in both 24 and 25 regions with both implants completely covered by regenerated bone (Fig. 7.10).[9,10]

Crestal Sinus Floor Elevation

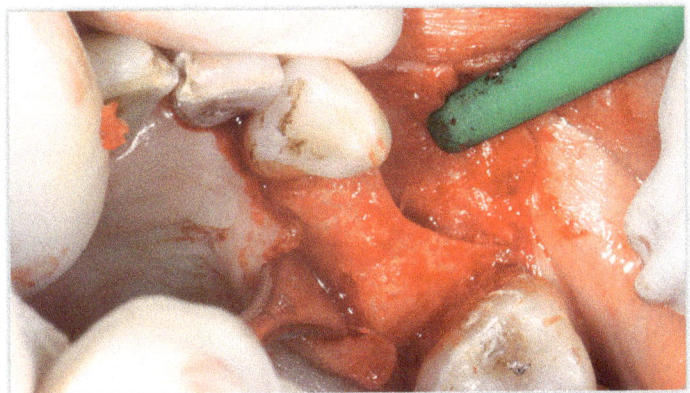

Fig. 7.5: Buccal concavity.

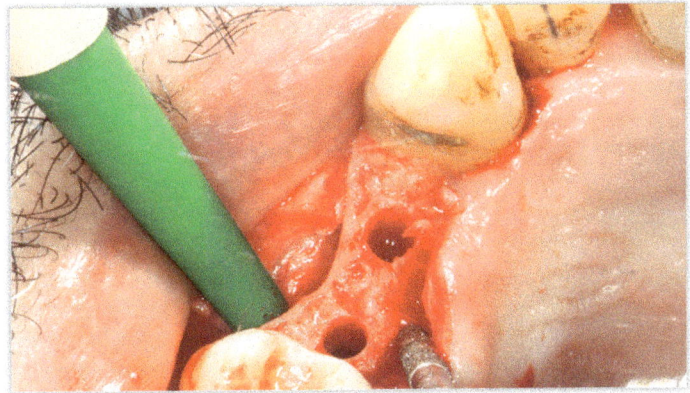

Fig. 7.6: Osteotomies prepared with intralift kit.

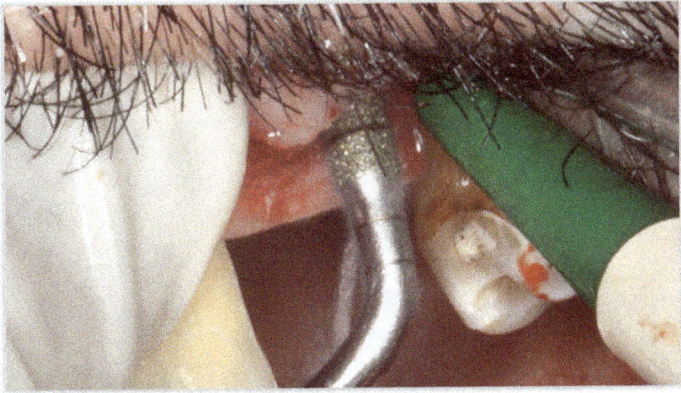

Fig. 7.7: Intralift TKW2 used to fracture sinus floor.

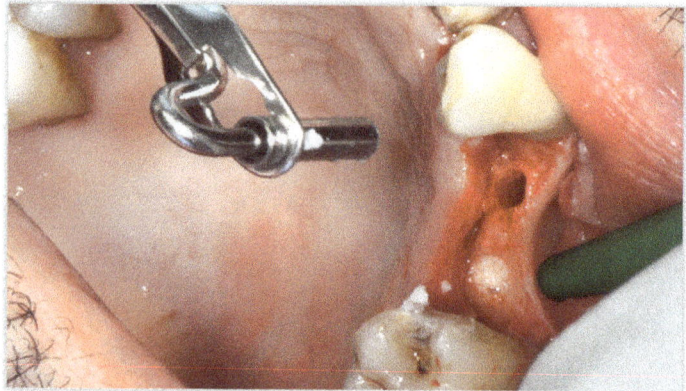

Fig. 7.8: Amalgam carrier used to introduce Bio-Oss into osteotomy site.

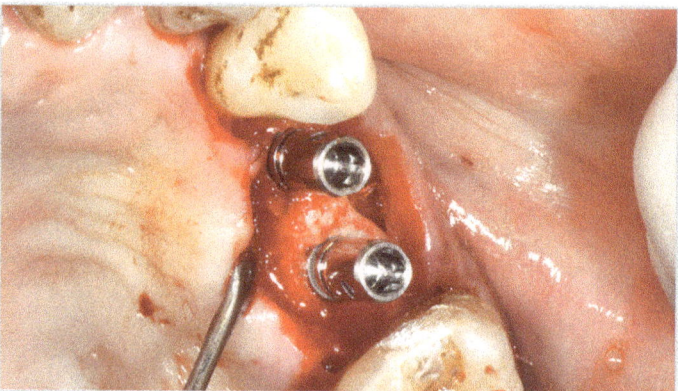

Fig. 7.9: Implants in place immediately after grafting.

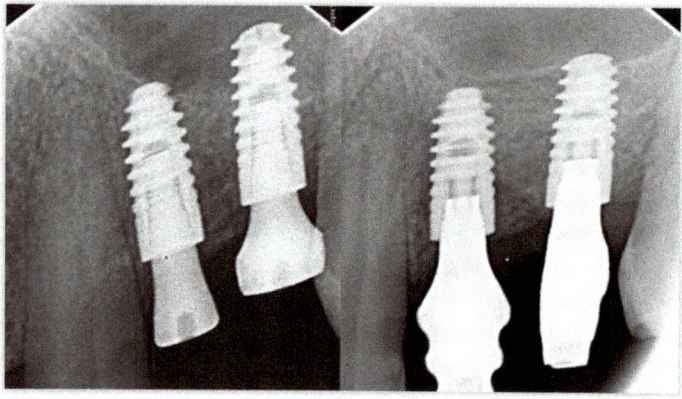

Fig. 7.10: Bone growth in the sinus cavity 6 months after grafting and implant placement.

CASE 2

Female aged 60 years presented with missing teeth nos 16 and 17. The width was sufficient for implant placement but the height in region 16 was only 2 mm and in region 17 was about 4 mm. In order to preserve the thin crestal bone, it was decided to do a flapless surgery. Flapless surgery has been shown to preserve the supraperiosteal blood supply to the bone which in-turn prevents alveolar crestal resorption.[11,12] After local anesthesia, a 4 mm wide motorized tissue punch was used (Fig. 7.11). The floor of the sinus was broken with the TKW2 (2.1 mm) after having used the TKW1 (1.6 mm) up to the floor of the sinus (Fig. 7.12). Subsequently, enlargement of the osteotomy was done with the TKW3 (2.35 mm) and TKW4 (2.8 mm). The TKW5 has a unique funnel-shaped tip with internal irrigation which is introduced right up to the floor of the sinus but not into the sinus cavity. The hydrodynamic pressure of the TKW5 internal irrigation at a reduced pressure of 70 was used to lift the sinus membrane evenly from lateral and medial surface for about 10 seconds this maneuver was repeated once again to be sure that the membrane was lifted from the floor of the sinus. In this case, Bio-Oss collagen (Geistlich) was used to graft the sinus cavity created by lifting the membrane. Bio-Oss collagen contains 90% Bio-Oss and 10% collagen with the result the particles of Bio-Oss are well integrated with the collagen and do not migrate, when placed in the sinus cavity (Fig. 7.13). The authors now prefer only Bio-Oss collagen for grafting the maxillary sinus cavity for either the crestal approach or the lateral approach because of its property of remaining in place and not migrating. Therefore even if undetected or inadvertently, there is perforation of the sinus membrane the Bio-Oss granules are prevented from migrating and closing the ostium and resultant congestion and possible sinusitis. Also Bio-Oss collagen can be broken into pieces and carried conveniently with tweezers into the osteotomy to be subsequently pushed first with the TKW4 (Fig. 7.14) and then with the TKW5 for ultrasonic and hydrodynamic compaction below the already lifted sinus membrane. Two Xive Implants (DentsplySirona) were next placed immediately. Xive 4.5/9.5 mm was placed in No. 16 and 4.5/11 mm

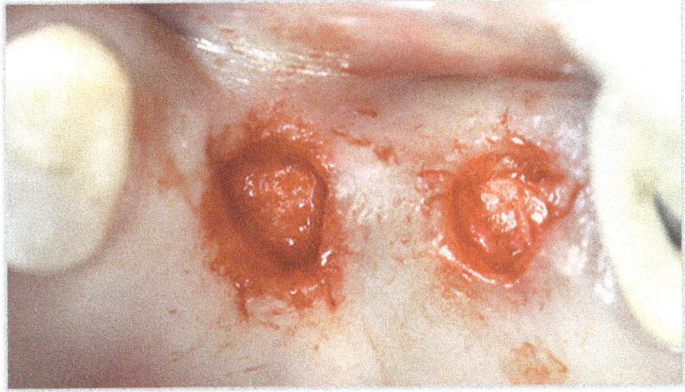

Fig. 7.11: Punched soft tissue after using motorized soft tissue punch.

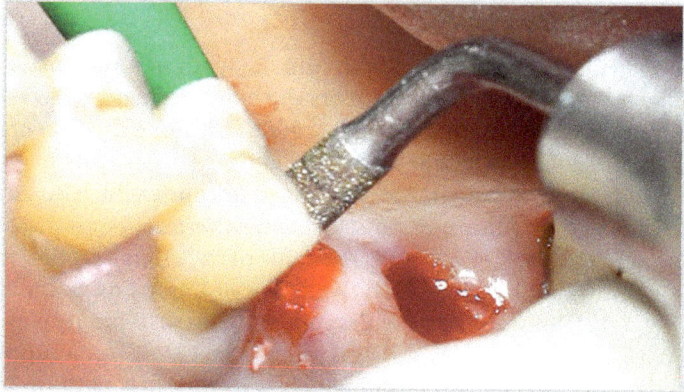

Fig. 7.12: TKW2 in use to fracture floor of sinus

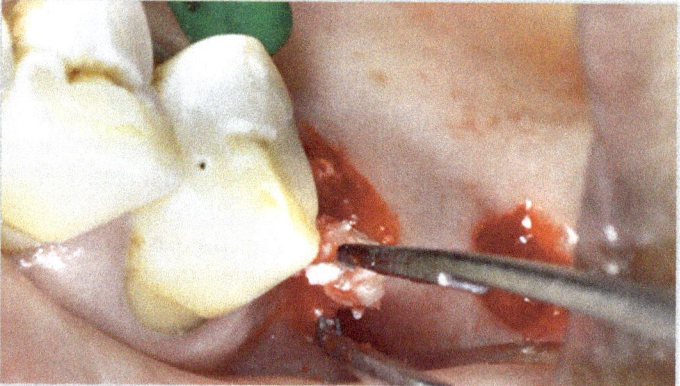

Fig. 7.13: Bio-Oss collagen introduced into osteotomy

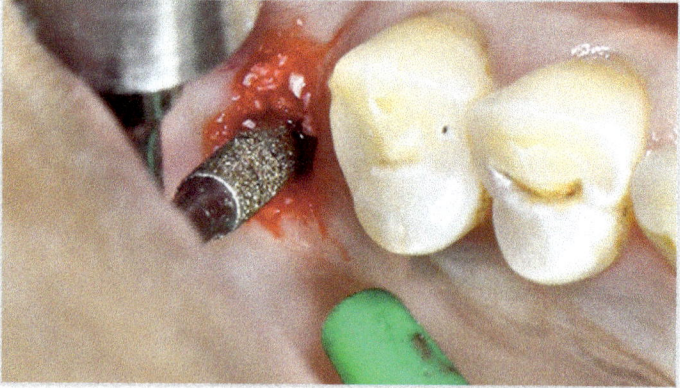

Fig. 7.14: TKW4 used to push the Bio-Oss Collagen towards floor of sinus.

was placed in 17 region with good primary stability. No drilling with the Xive drills was done. The self-tapping capability of the Xive implants allowed us to do this. Also the poor bone quality in the posterior maxilla allows undersizing of implant site. In case where the quality of bone is good you may have to use the 3.4 and 3.8 mm Xive drill before placement of the 4.5 mm implant. However, when using the drills extreme care must be taken to prevent entering into the sinus cavity with the drills. An IOPA immediately after placement of implants confirms correct placement and Bio-Oss collagen material all-round the implants (Fig. 7.15). The implants were left transmucosal with 2 mm gingival formers. Eight months of healing was allowed instead of the usual 6 months because of poor quality of bone and also since we had only 2 mm of height of bone in 16 region. CBCT taken at 8 months shows gain of bone height of about 7 mm in 16 and 17 regions, also apex of the implants are covered by bone (Fig. 7.16) Cross-sectional comparison of the CBCT before placement and grafting of implants with CBCT taken after 8 months, clearly confirm growth of bone of 7 mm (Fig. 7.17).

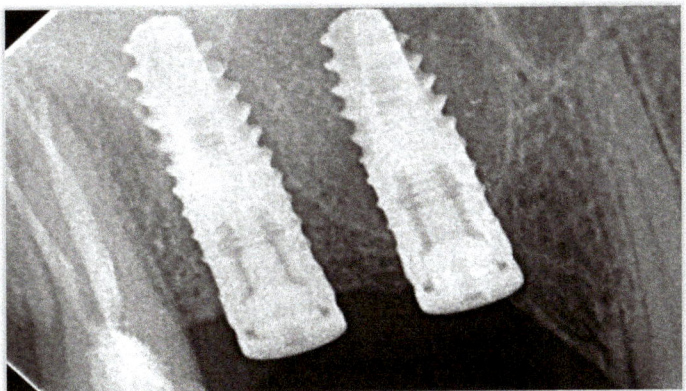

Fig. 7.15: IOPA taken on day of surgery.

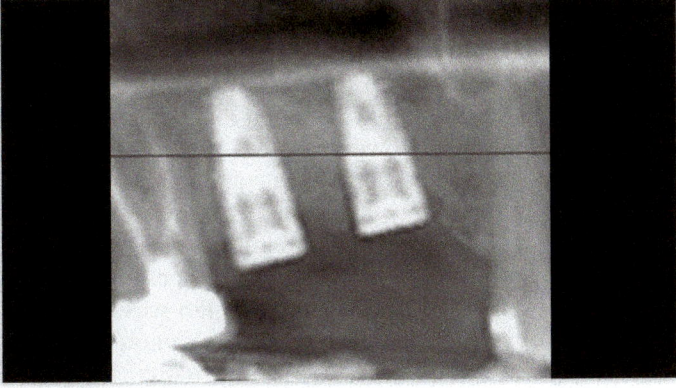

Fig. 7.16: Panoramic view of CBCT after 8 months.

104 Clinical Guide to Oral Implantology: Step by Step Procedures

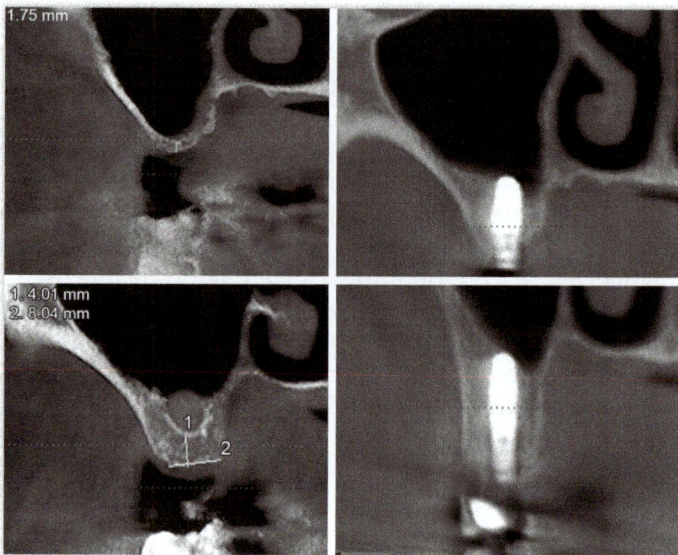

Fig. 7.17: Comparison of CBCTs before grafting and placement of implants and after 8 months of healing period.

CASE 3

A 65-year-old male patient whose extraction of tooth number 27 was done 7 months ago wishes to now replace the missing tooth with implant supported fixed restoration instead of a 3 unit fixed bridge. CBCT taken after 7 months of bone healing reveals a crestal height of about 6mm from floor of sinus and a width of about 9 mm. It was therefore decided to do a flapless sinus floor elevation and grafting. However, this time instead of using Bio-Oss collagen which was not available in India at that time, it was decided to mix particulate Bio-Oss granules small size and mix it with autologous fibrin glue made by centrifuging of patients own venous blood (Fig. 7.18). For details of this technique, readers may refer the original work by Choukran and/or by Dong-Seok Sohn[8]. Although data is not robust about platelet-derived growth factors (PDGF) from patients own venous blood in accelerating regeneration of hard and soft tissues, some studies are available but more research is needed before it can be definitely concluded that it plays a major role in hard and soft tissue regeneration. However even if it does not play a major role in bone regeneration autologous fibrin glue agglomerates and makes Bio-Oss sticky which acts like Bio-Oss collagen and prevents migration and blocking the ostium in case of perforation of the membrane (Fig. 7.19). After the sinus membrane had been elevated using the same technique as described in Case 2. Sticky bone instead of Bio-Oss collagen was introduced into the osteotomy and subsequently carried and compacted below the raised membrane using the funnel shaped and internally irrigated TKW5. After

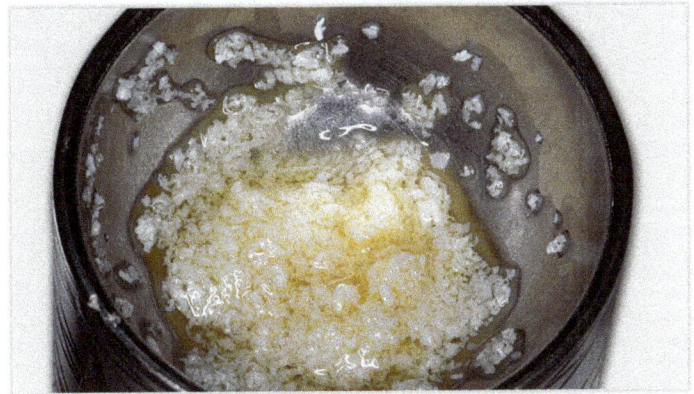

Fig. 7.18: Preparation of sticky bone.

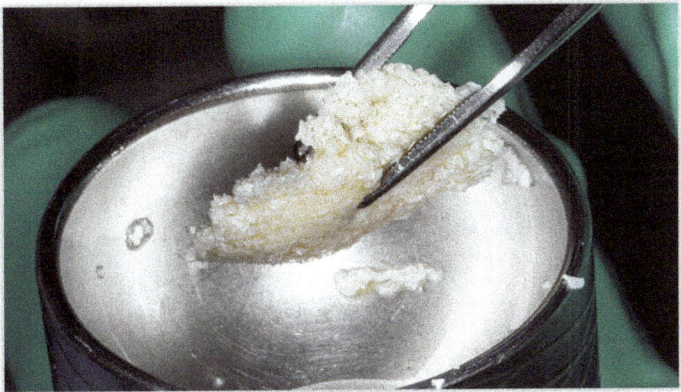

Fig. 7.19: Sticky bone behaves such as Bio-Oss Collagen with added advantage of growth factors.

compacting the sticky bone underneath, the membrane platelet rich fibrin (PRF) membrane was introduced into the sinus cavity before placement of Xive 4.5/13 mm implant (DentsplySirona) with excellent primary stability (Fig. 7.20). IOPA and CBCT was taken immediately after implant placement shows grafted sticky bone covering apex of the implant. Implant were not submerged but were left to heal transmucosally with gingival formers (Fig. 7.21). CBCT taken after six months of healing shows replacement of sticky bone with newly regenerated bone and obliteration of the old cortical demarcation of the sinus floor. After progressive bone loading for 6 weeks with a composite crown, a definitive full contour zirconia crown was delivered and cemented with resin modified glass ionomer cement (RelyX luting cement 3M ESPE).

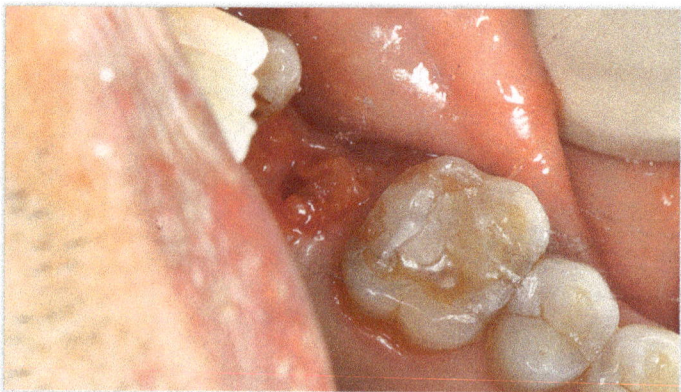

Fig. 7.20: Xive (Dentsply Sirona) implants in place.

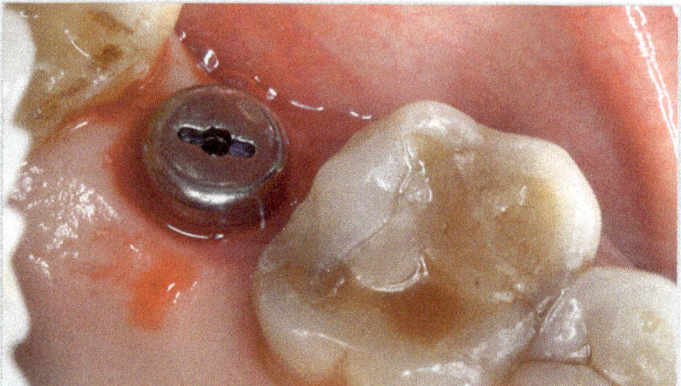

Fig. 7.21: Transmucosal healing with gingival formers.

REFERENCES

1. Watzek G, Ulm CW, Haas R. Anatomic and physiologic fundamentals of sinus floor augmentation. In: Jensen OT, (Ed): The Sinus Bone Graft. Chicago, Ill: Quintessence; 1999:31-47.
2. Boyne PJ, James RA. Grafting of the maxillary sinus floor with autogenous marrow and bone. J Oral Surg. 1980;38:613-6.
3. Summers RB. A new concept in maxillary implant surgery: The osteotome technique. Compendium. 1994;15:152, 154-6, 158.
4. Woo I, Le BT. Maxillary sinus floor elevation: Review of anatomy and two techniques. Implant Dent 2004;13:28-32

5. Saker M, Ogle O. Benign paroxysmal positional vertigo subsequent to sinus lift via closed technique. J Oral Maxillofac Surg. 2005, 63:1385-87.
6. Rosen PS, Summers R, Mellado JR, Salkin LM, Shanaman RH, Marks MH, Fugazzotto PA. The bone-added osteotome sinus floor elevation technique: multicenter retrospective report of consecutively treated patients. Int J Oral Maxillofac Implants. 1999;14(6):853-8.
7. Vercellotti T. Piezoelectric surgery in implantology: a case report—a new piezoelectric ridge expansion technique. Int J Periodontics Restorative Dent. 2000;20:358–65.
8. Sohn DS, Lee JS, An KM, et al. Piezoelectric internal sinus elevation (PISE) technique: A new method for internal sinus elevation. Implant Dent. 2009;18: 458–63.
9. Romanos, George E. Nentwig, George-Hubertus. Immediate functional loading in the maxilla using implants with platform switching: Five-year results. Int J Oral Maxillofac Implants. 2009; 24(6): 1106-12.
10. Dibart S, Warbington M, Su MF, Skobe Z. *In vitro* evaluation of the implant-abutment bacterial seal: the locking taper system. Int J Oral Maxillofac Implants. 2005; 20(5):732-7.
11. Pfeifer JS. The reaction of alveolar bone to flap procedures in man. Periodontic. 1965: 3:135-40
12. Chen ST, Darby IB, Reynolds EC, Clement JG. Immediate implant placement postextraction without flap elevation. J Periodontol. 2009;80(1):163-72.

Chapter 8

Immediate Implantation and Provisionalization in the Anterior Maxilla

Implant placement immediately after extraction followed by an immediate provisional restoration can be a very rewarding way to provide implant therapy to our patients (Box 8.1). It provides significant benefit both to the patient and the dentist compared with traditional delayed protocol of waiting for 4–6 months. The procedure also reduces the number of surgeries which may be beneficial both to the dentist and the patient. Factors critical to success include good initial implant primary stability in good quality bone. It is generally, (however not always) avoided when the labial plate of bone is missing and grafting is required. Immediate implant placement and loading is technically challenging and should only be undertaken by clinicians with considerable experience with implant dentistry, both surgically and prosthetically.

CRESTAL BONE LOSS AND THE BIOLOGIC WIDTH

Preservation of crestal bone after 2 stage implant placement has been a concern. Because of the importance of bone to aesthetics, the postoperative reduction of crestal bone after 2 stage implant therapy needs to be addressed. Crestal bone loss results in recession of the gingival margins and sometimes the papilla, particularly in individuals with thin biotypes.[1]

The manner in which the junctional epithelium and connective tissue attaches to the tooth and to the implant differ. Whilst the junctional epithelium attaches by way of glycoproteins to the natural dentition, a pseudo attachment through hemidesmosomes exists around endosseous implants. In addition, connective tissue fibres mechanically insert into natural root cementum whereas in the case of implants, a tight cuff of connective tissue is formed around the titanium implant.

BOX 8.1: Advantages of immediate implant placement into extraction sockets and provisional restorations.

- Immediate aesthetics by a fixed restoration
- Prevents collapse of the peri-implant soft tissue through support given by a carefully crafted provisional restoration
- Reduces the number of surgeries
- Reduces time required for rehabilitation

Gargiulo[2] documented a biologic width from the base of the gingival sulcus to the crest of the alveolar bone to be 2.04 mm, with epithelial attachment of 0.97 mm and connective tissue attachment of 1.07 mm. The dimensions in implants are supposed to be similar to those of natural teeth and are stable even after loading. These dimensions are a key determinant of aesthetics.

Following abutment connection, the crestal bone loss has been shown to recede from the implant abutment connection by 1.3 to 1.4 mm. However, with certain implant systems like 'ANKYLOS' (Dentsply Sirona Implants Germany) which employ platform switching and a strong conical implant abutment connection, this crestal bone loss at stage 2 surgery is nearly eliminated. The 'ANKYLOS' system in the mid 1980's was one of the first systems to introduce the morse taper conical connection with platform switching of the implant abutment connection. Some of the other companies who have similar features are AstraTech Dentsply Sirona Implants, Sweden; Bicon, Boston; Curasan, Germany, Nobel Active, Nobel Biocare; and Straumann BL, Switzerland. The 'ANKYLOS' system is unique because it not only has platform switching which brings the bacterial inflammatory infiltrate from the bone towards the axis of the implant but more important the very strong conical implant abutment connection has no microgaps and also prevents micromovements resulting in no bacterial colonization. This unique combination of platform switching and strong implant abutment connection has been documented since the last 23 years to virtually eliminate crestal bone loss which in turn preserves soft tissue architecture. The preservation of the peri-implant bone is particularly important in the aesthetic zone where the objective is to prevent post- prosthetic bone loss and preserve soft tissues. The 'ANKYLOS' implant system is also grit blasted and thermally acid etched right up to the shoulder of the implant with no polished collar which encourage the bone to grow right up to the top of the implant thus allowing 1 mm sub-crestal placement of the implant. Implants with smooth collars when placed subcrestally, the bone resorbs all the way down to the rough to smooth transition line.

Immediate placement and providing a customized immediate provisional restoration with appropriate subgingival emergence profile can be of significant benefit in providing stability to the peri-implant soft tissues. Careful manipulations of the hard and soft tissues are critical to a successful outcome of the procedure. Extractions should be done as atraumatically as possible with microsurgical blades, periotomes and luxators taking care not to injure or fracture the labial cortical plate of bone. Intrasulcular incisions and minimal or no reflection of the periosteum (flapless procedure) should be employed.[3]

Although, implant placement into fresh extraction sockets is now considered to be a predictable and accepted treatment procedure, there are important prerequisites for immediate implantation which must be addressed (Box 8.2).

In the maxillary aesthetic zone, implant placement should be undertaken towards the palatal aspect of the extraction socket and one should not follow the same direction of the extraction socket (Fig. 8.1). Care must be taken during the osteotomy preparation on the palatal wall, as this is dense and difficult to prepare.

BOX 8.2: Prerequisites for immediate implantation.
- Adequate primary stability
- Adequate bone all around the implant covering and stabilizing the implant
- Preferably no grafting procedure needs to be undertaken especially no major grafting. If extensive grafting has to be done, implant should be submerged, wait for bone and implant to osseointegrate, before loading
- No major infection or soft tissue inflammation should be present. Small periapical granulomas are not a contraindication as they can be eliminated by surgical curetting and subsequent osteotomy
- Sufficient bone apically to ensure primary stability.

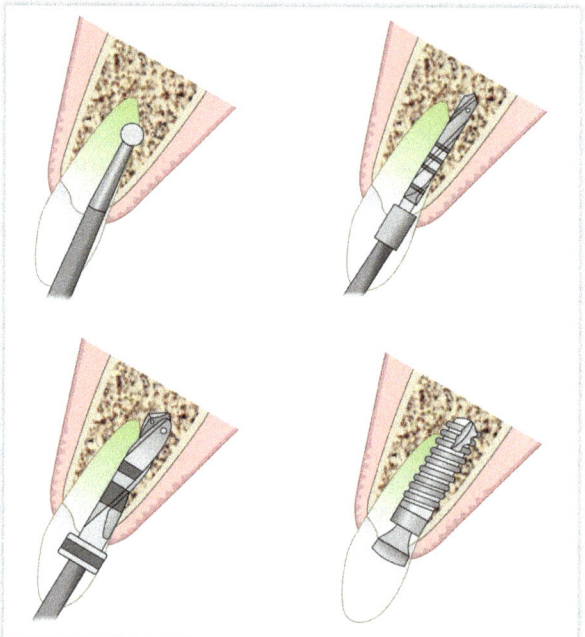

Fig. 8.1: Initial drilling into the apical part of palatal bone, followed by incremental sizing of osteotomy with Lindemann and final twist drill. Resulting in proper 3D placement of Implant.

If immediate provisional restoration is considered, it is essential to have about 35 Ncm of insertion torque. If moderate primary stability of about 25 Ncm is achieved, then a transmucosal healing screw can be placed to avoid second stage surgery. If, however, there is poor primary stability with less than 20 Ncm, then it is advisable to place cover screws and submerge the implant and wait for osseointegration (3–4 months) before loading the implant. The purpose of the following case reports is to further explain and elucidate the concept of immediate implantation and provisionalization.

CASE 1

A female aged 46 years, the CEO of a multinational company fractured the crown off from her upper right first premolar and was faced with an embarrassing situation because the tooth gap was visible when she smiled. She requested an immediate aesthetic solution with a fixed restoration (Figs. 8.2 and 8.3). Looking to the emergency of the situation, the treatment plan was to extract the remaining root and place an implant immediately with non-functional loading, this plan according to us would be the most conservative (no reduction of adjacent natural teeth) and long lasting method of rehabilitation. On an emergency basis, the next day; after the usual preoperative investigations and medications, the roots were atraumatically removed using first the no.15C blade to sever the periodontal fibers (Fig. 8.4) followed by the periotome (Fig. 8.5) and finally using the very thin luxator (Fig. 8.6). Only after the root was mobile, was the straight root forceps used to remove the roots (Fig. 8.7). There were two

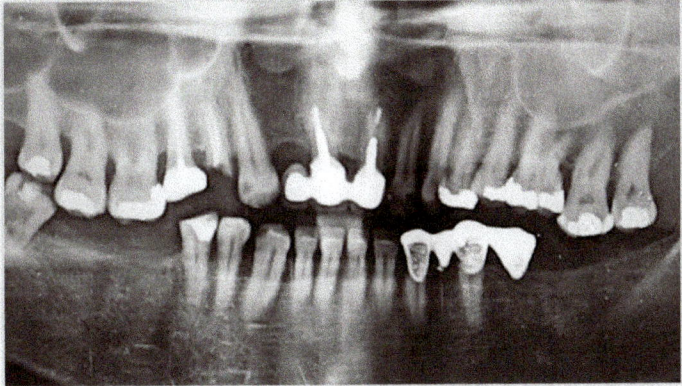

Fig. 8.2: Preoperative orthopantomogram (OPG).

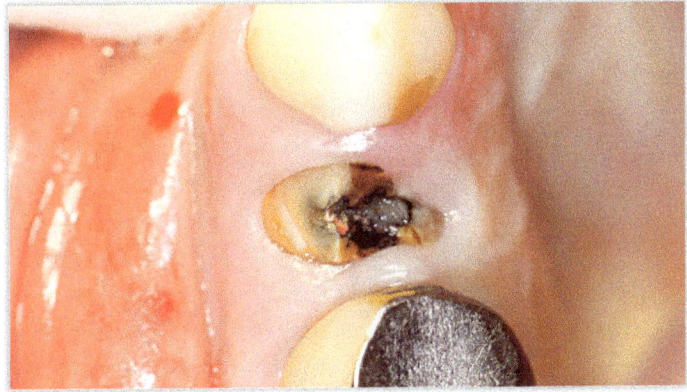

Fig. 8.3: Intraoral view of fractured tooth.

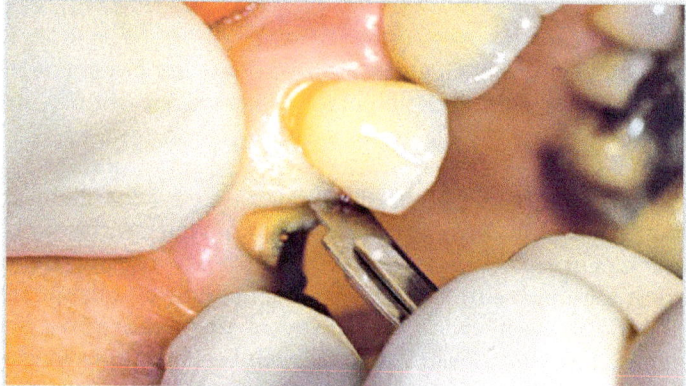

Fig. 8.4: Use of no.15 blade to sever the periodontal fibers.

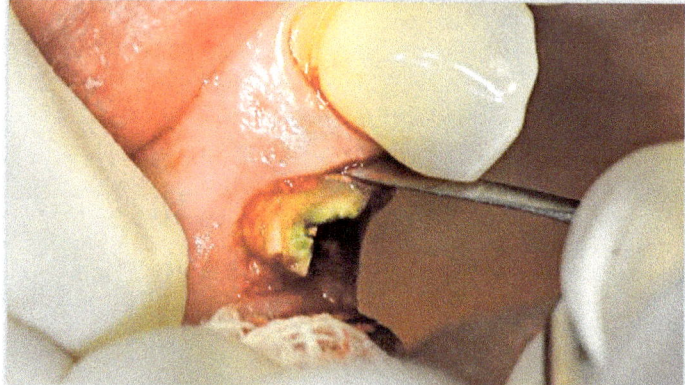

Fig. 8.5: Subsequent use of periotome to sever and widen the periodontal membrane space.

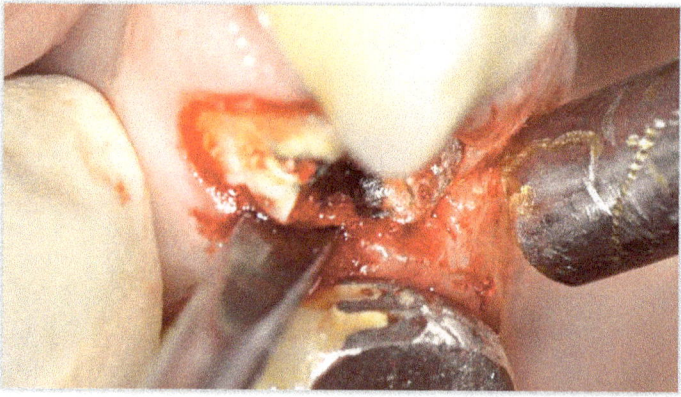

Fig. 8.6: Use of luxator on the mesial and distal surface.

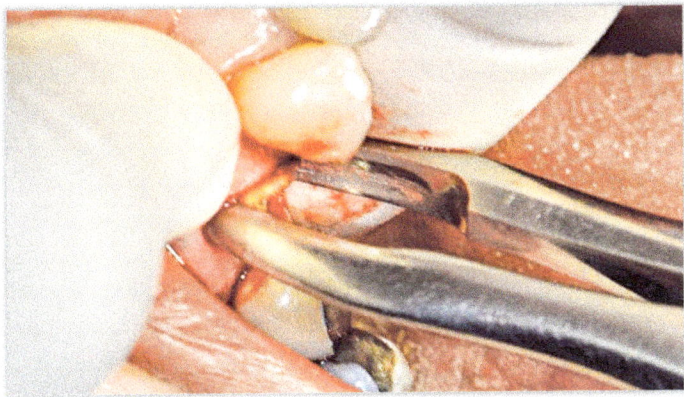

Fig. 8.7: Use of forcep only after tooth is mobile.

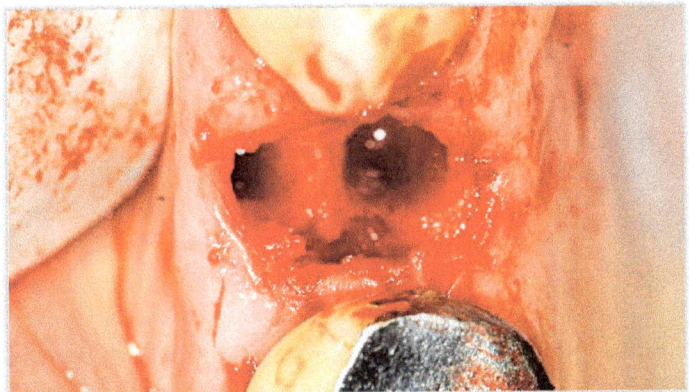

Fig. 8.8: Intraoral view of extraction socket.

separate roots with a clear septa (Fig. 8.8). It was decided to use the 'ANKYLOS' Implant system because of its established 'tissue care' concept of preserving crestal bone and in turn soft tissue around the implants (Figs. 8.9 and 8.10).

It was also decided to use the 'ANKYLOS' Balance Abutment (Fig. 8.11) at the time of surgery itself and modify it extraorally. The advantage of placing the final abutment at the time of surgery, avoids the need to change abutments and in turn preserves the bone and soft tissue. The precaution to take is to only torque the abutment with hand pressure at the time of surgery. The final torquing with the wrench should be undertaken after osseointegration, i.e. minimum of two months. With the 'Plus' surface of the 'ANKYLOS' implants which is treated right up to the shoulder of the implant, accelerated hard and soft tissue integration is achieved (Figs. 8.12 to 8.15).

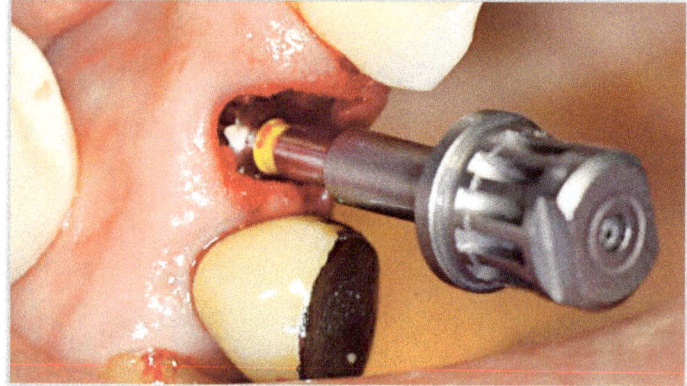

Fig. 8.9: Conical reamer prepares the osteotomy to the final shape and more importantly, is an indicator of the primary stability of the implant.

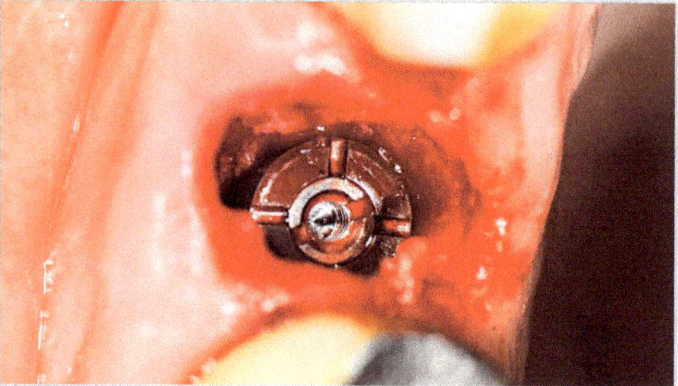

Fig. 8.10: Final placement of the implant 3 mm below the free gingival margin and about 1 mm subcrestally.

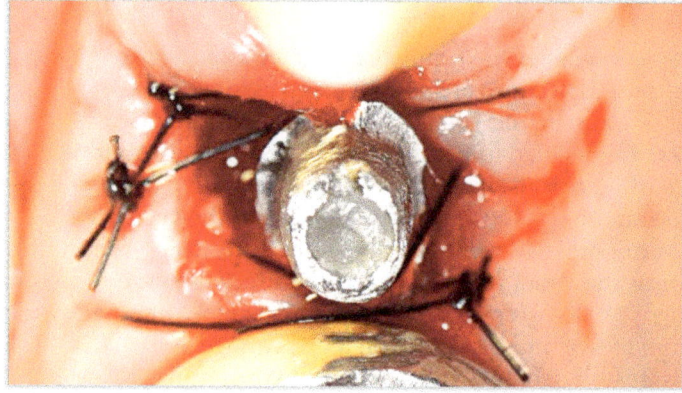

Fig. 8.11: Modified abutment torqued in by hand and access hole sealed with temporary elastic composite.

Immediate Implantation and Provisionalization in the Anterior Maxilla

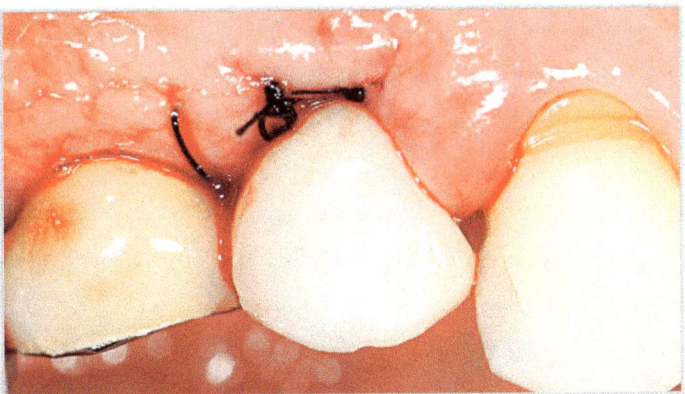

Fig. 8.12: Temporary crown cemented with non-eugenol temporary cement Temp Bond NE (Kerr) at the time of surgery.

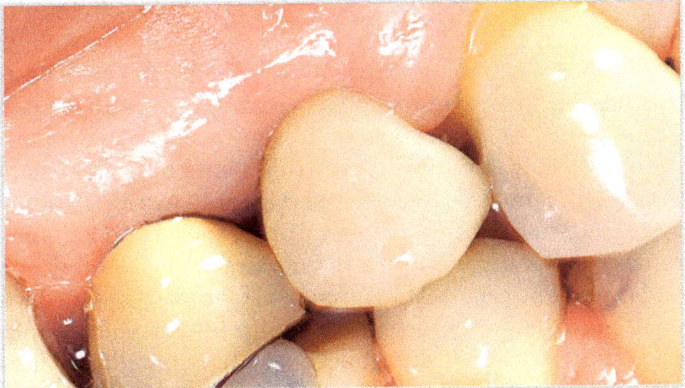

Fig. 8.13: Temporary crown after one month without any modification. Note: The excellent healing and support of the hard and soft tissues because of the morse taper connection of the "Ankylos" implant system.

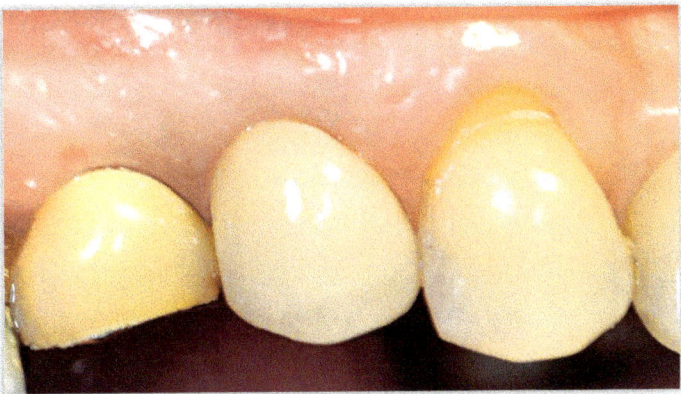

Fig. 8.14: Final porcelain-fused-to-metal (PFM) crown after 3 months post-surgery.

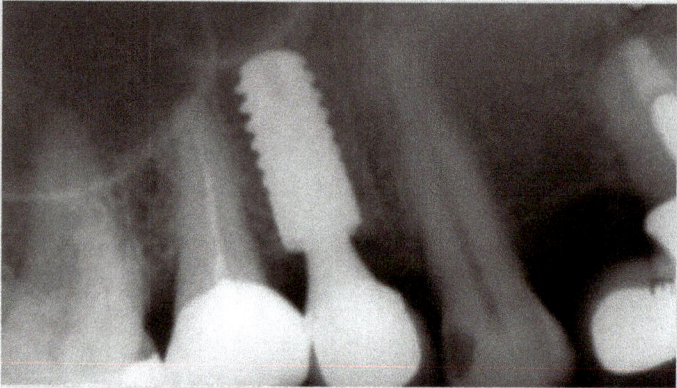

Fig. 8.15: Final intraoral radiograph before cementation of crown.

CASE 2

Male aged 34 years presents with fractured central incisor which had a post and core (Fig. 8.16). He requested immediate restoration of his aesthetics with a fixed restoration. The treatment plan in consultation with the patient was to do an extraction, immediate implantation and provisionalization.

The tooth was atraumatically extracted using periotomes and luxators preserving the thin buccal plate of bone (Figs. 8.17 to 8.19). Drilling was done in the apical one-third of the palatal wall of the socket and implant osteotomy was prepared palatally without causing any pressure on the thin buccal cortical plate of bone (Fig. 8.20). The conical reamer was placed with the help of Nentwig's instrument holder which confirmed the correct apico-coronal, mesiodistal and very importantly buccopalatal preparation of the osteotomy (Fig. 8.21). With the help of the motor, the implant was placed at a speed of 15 rpm and a torque of 45 Ncm, care was taken to see that it was placed 3 mm below the free gingival margin (Figs. 8.22 and 8.23). The cover screw was removed and a balance straight abutment with a gingival height of 3 mm was torqued in by hand pressure (Figs. 8.24A and B). An impression in Aquasil Soft

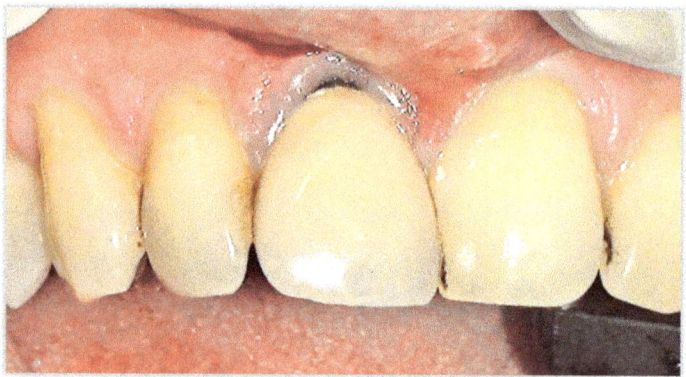

Fig. 8.16: Preoperative view of non-salvageable upper right central incisor.

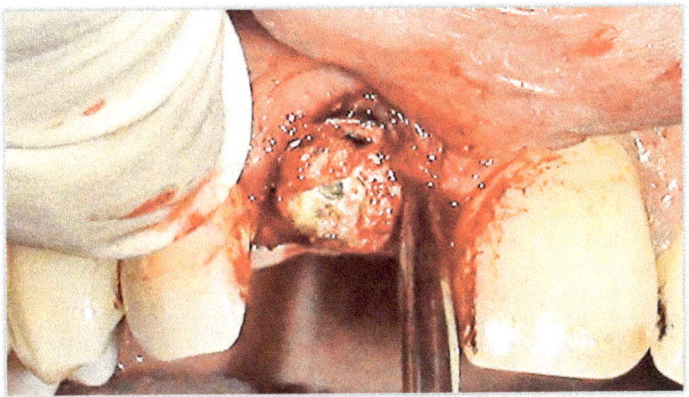

Fig. 8.17: Atraumatic luxation of the fractured root.

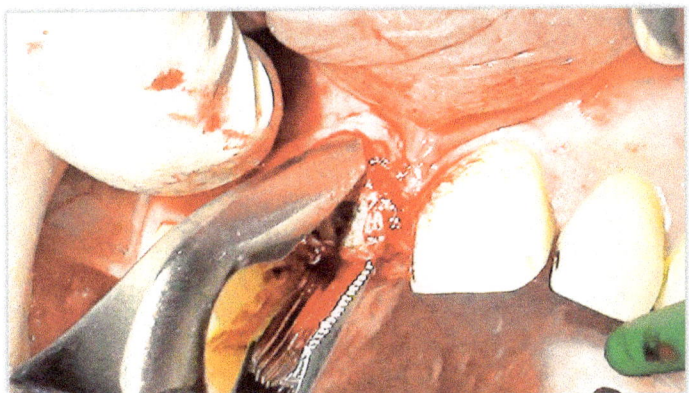

Fig. 8.18: Removal of the luxated root by rotational movements of the root forcep.

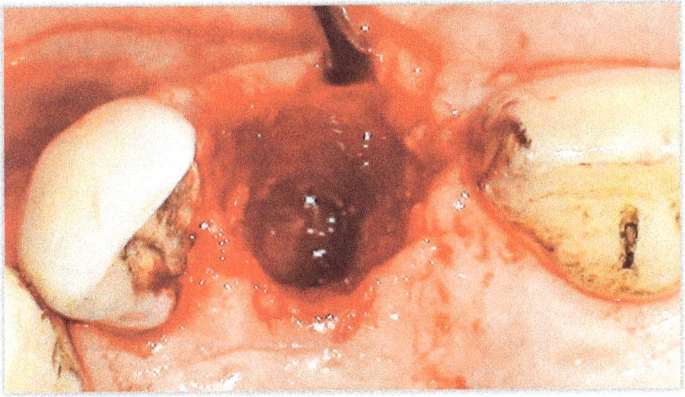

Fig. 8.19: Intact buccal plate of bone was preserved.

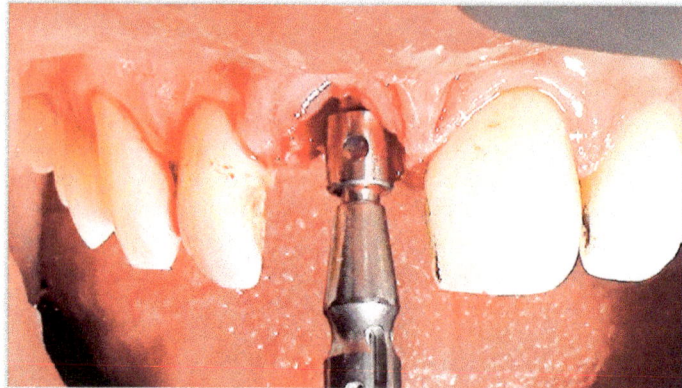

Fig. 8.20: 2 mm twist drill with drill extension.

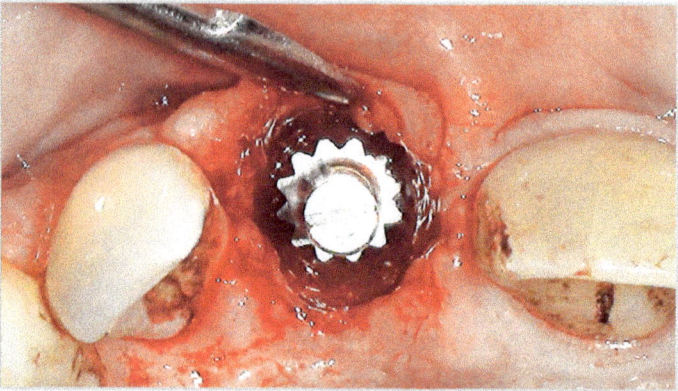

Fig. 8.21: Conical reamer confirms correct three-dimensional preparation of osteotomy.

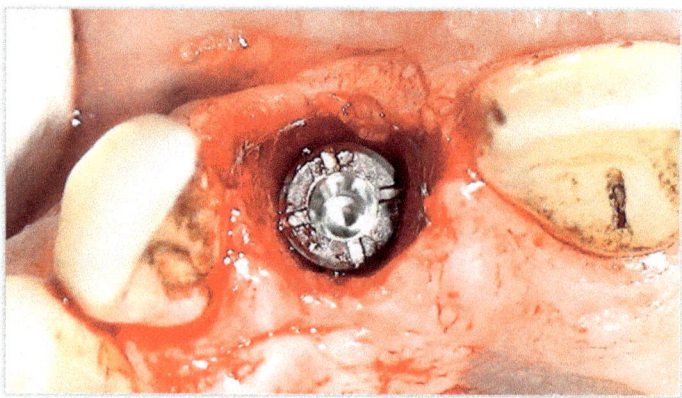

Fig. 8.22: Ankylos B/11 implant placed resting against the palatal cortical bone.

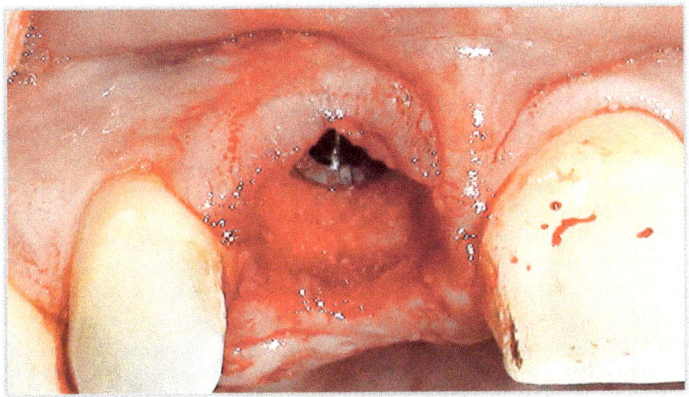

Fig. 8.23: Correct apico-coronal placement of implant, 3 mm from free gingival margin.

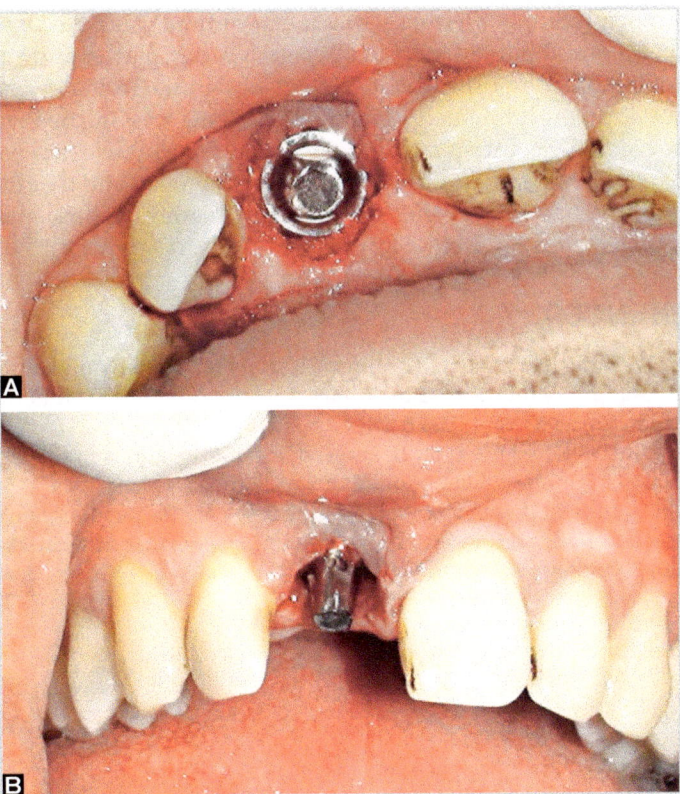

Figs. 8.24A and B: Balance abutment 3.0 GH, straight was torqued in by hand pressure.

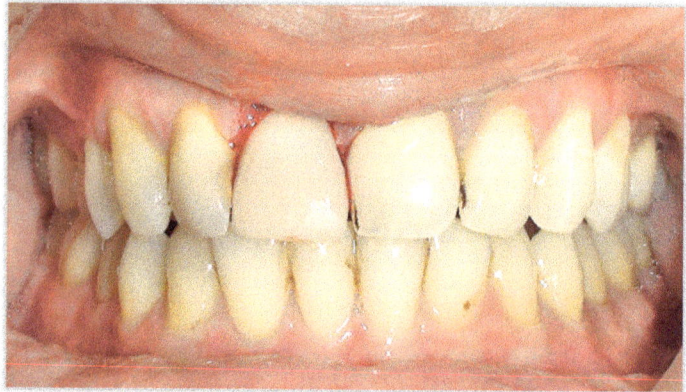

Fig. 8.25: Provisional composite crown cemented with non-eugenol temporary cement.

Putty (Dentsply Sirona, Germany) was taken without using the Light Viscosity. A cast was poured immediately in fast setting stone plaster and a provisional using sculptable composite Ceram-x (Dentsply Sirona Germany) was prepared in the clinic on the lubricated stone cast. The same was finished and polished and provisionally cemented with a non-eugenol cement. Care was taken to see that all the excess temporary cement was removed and that there was no contact of the provisional with the opposing teeth in centric and eccentric movements of the mandible (Fig. 8.25).

REFERENCES

1. Kan JY, Rungcharassaeng K, Umezu K, Kois JC. Dimensions of peri-implant mucosa: an evaluation of maxillary anterior single implants in humans. J Periodontol. 2003;74(4):558.62.
2. Gargiulo A, Wentz F, Orban B. Dimensions and Relations of the Dentogingival Junction in Humans. J Periodontol. 1961;32:261-8.
3. Fickl S, Zuhr O, Wachtel H, Bolz W, Huerzeler M. Tissue alterations after tooth extraction with and without surgical trauma: a volumetric study in the beagle dog. J Clin Periodontol. 2008;35(4):356-63.

Chapter 9

Implant Aesthetics

The premaxilla is a highly aesthetic zone. It often requires both hard (bone and teeth) and soft tissue management. The soft tissue drape is often the most difficult to restore. The anterior single tooth restoration is therefore the greatest challenge even for the most experienced and skillful practitioner. There are major difficulties in placing the implants because of the various local risk factors that can compromise the final aesthetic outcome (Table 9.1).

From our experience, the following criteria are important to prevent loss of hard and soft tissue to achieve optimum aesthetics:
- All attempts should be made to place an implant immediately after extraction and definitely not more than four weeks after extraction, to minimize resorption of the labial plate of bone.
- Extraction should be carried out with minimal damage to the bone and soft tissues. The use of microsurgical blades, periotomes (Medesy, Associated Dental, Mumbai) and finally very thin luxators (Directa, Sweden) is recommended (Figs. 9.1A to C).
- Correct 3D placement of the implant should be achieved, especially in the buccopalatal region, taking care not to touch the fragile buccal plate. It is not necessary to fill the complete socket buccopalatally with a larger diameter implant, rather a space may be left labially, which can be grafted with slow resorbing bovine bone mineral (Fig. 9.2)
- Implants should be tapered with a progressive thread design, i.e. the implant threads get progressively deeper towards the apical end engaging more bone in the soft spongy area in the apical region. This ensures primary stability even in a compromised bone. However, for implant success its crestal part should have shallower threads to prevent excessive stress in the dense cortical bone of the region (Fig. 9.3).

TABLE 9.1: Hurdles in placing implants in the pre-maxillary zone.
- High incidence of missing labial plate of bone.
- High potential loss of interdental papillae leading to black triangles.
- Less than optimal bone quality.

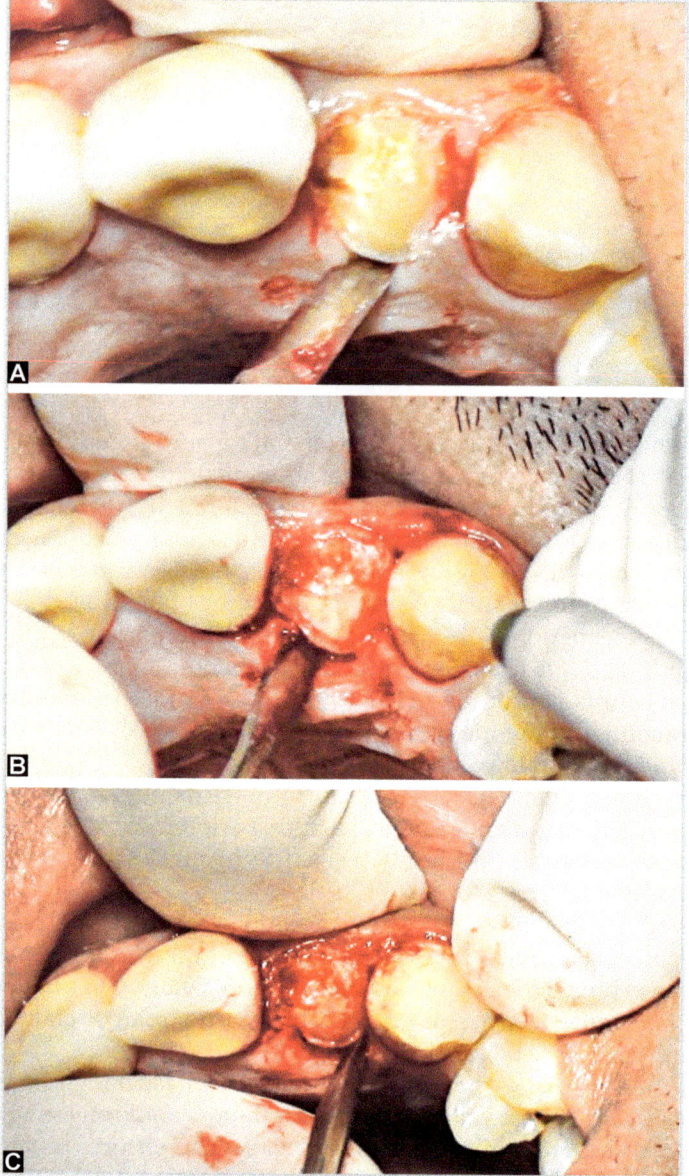

Figs. 9.1A to C: (A) Atraumatic extraction of the tooth starting with microsurgical No.15 blade followed by periotome in (B), and finally a thin luxator in (C). The periotomes and luxators should apply pressure on the mesiodistal surfaces and palatal surfaces only. The microsurgical blade maybe used to severe the periodontal ligament fibers on the labial aspect.

Implant Aesthetics

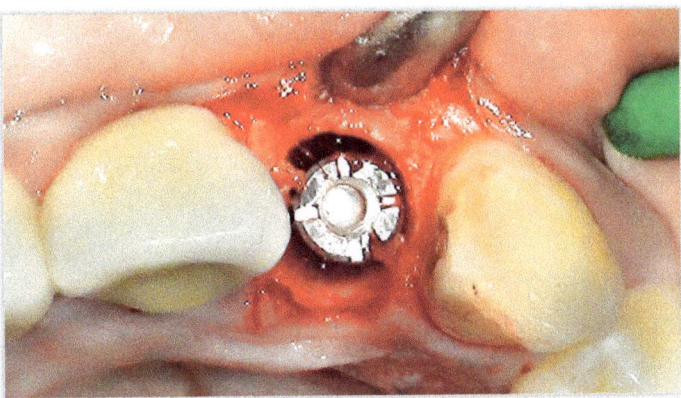

Fig. 9.2: Correct labiopalatal placement of the implant in the extraction socket with space of about 2–3 mm on the labial aspect, which maybe grafted with particulate mineral bovine bone.

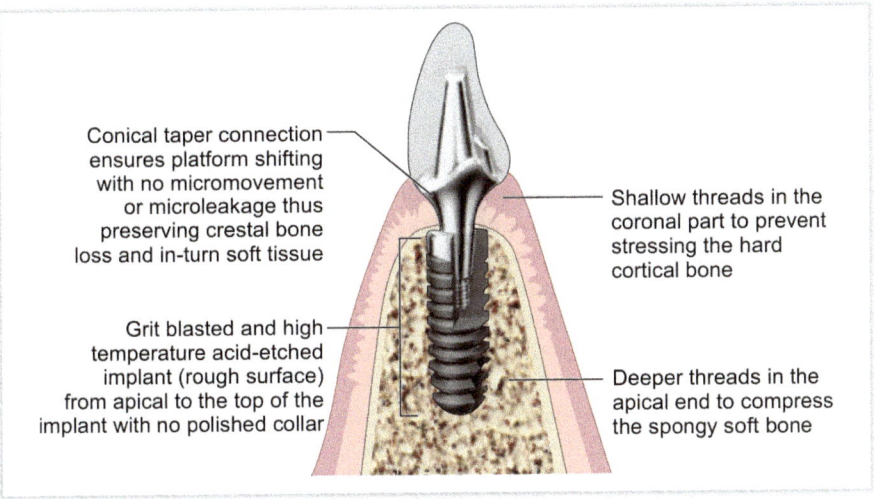

Fig. 9.3: The unique "ANKYLOS" implant (Dentsply Sirona, Germany) with progressive thread design and conical-tapered connection.

- Implants should not have any polished collar and should be surface treated (roughened) right up to the platform. This results in minimal bone loss during remodeling[1,2] (Figs. 9.3 and 9.4)
- The implant abutment connection should be a conical tapered one to prevent micromovement and microleakage. This will be helpful for stability of the peri-implant hard and soft tissues[3] (Fig. 9.3).

To better understand the concepts outlined above to achieve optimum aesthetics, the following case report is presented.

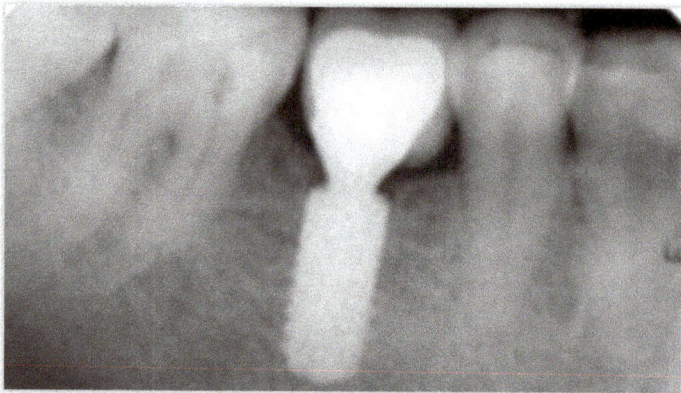

Fig. 9.4: Although the implant is placed subcrestally, observe the excellent preservation of the crestal bone. Implant in service since last 2 years.

CASE REPORT

Patient aged 54 years comes with a complaint of pain, swelling and grade III mobility in the region of upper right central incisor (Figs. 9.5A and B). Patient was given an option of endodontics combined with periodontic treatment with a guarded prognosis or extraction, immediate implantation and provisionalisation. He opted for the latter treatment.

Subsequently the tooth was extracted and thorough curettage of the apical area as well as the remaining bony walls was done. With the precision drill (Power Point Drill Laxmi Associates, Bangaluru), a purchase point was made in the apical end of the palatal wall (Fig. 9.6). Next, the Lindemann drill was used to enlarge the osteotomy and to partially counter sink into the palatal wall. This was followed by the 2 mm twist drill to a depth of 14 mm. Incrementally, the osteotomy was enlarged to the 4.5 mm twist drill at the expense of the palatal wall. The conical reamer was used to check the stability and the correct depth of the osteotomy (Figs. 9.7 and 9.8). The bone was tapped to full length. The implant was placed with the motor at 45 N-cm torque with firm pressure against the palatal wall in order to prevent the apical part of the implant from drifting labially (Fig. 9.9). The cover screw was removed and an Ankylos balance abutment with a gingival height of 3 mm and at an angulation of 15° was torqued in by hand (Figs. 9.10 and 9.11). The impression of the abutment was taken with Aquasil putty only without using the light viscosity. A cast was poured immediately in fast-setting stone plaster and a provisional using sculptable composite Ceram-x (Dentsply DeTrey Germany) was prepared in the clinic on the lubricated stone cast. The same was finished and polished and provisionally cemented with a non-eugenol cement (Fig. 9.12). Care was taken to see that all the excess temporary cement was removed and that there was no contact of the provisional with the opposing teeth in centric and eccentric movements of the mandible (Fig. 9.13).

Implant Aesthetics

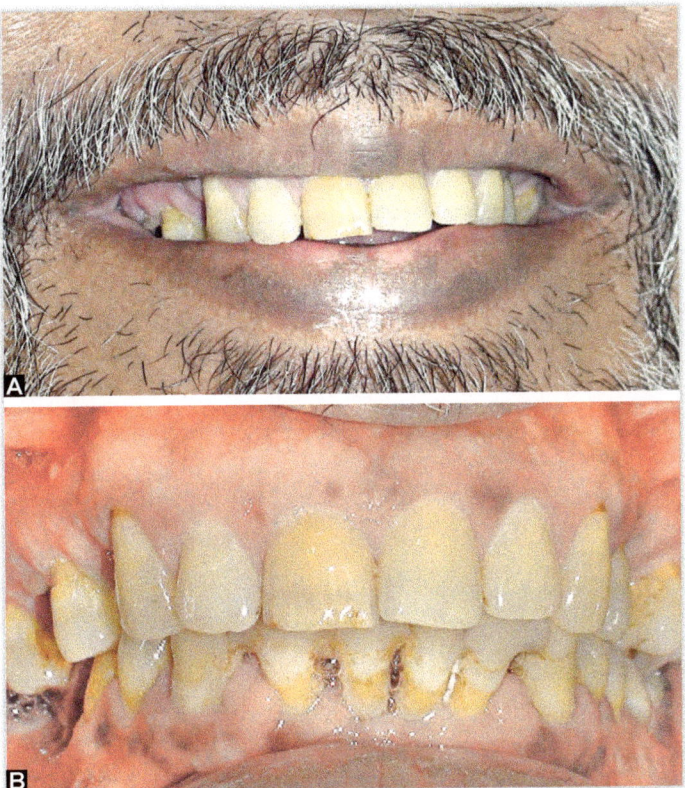

Figs. 9.5A and B: Preoperative photographs

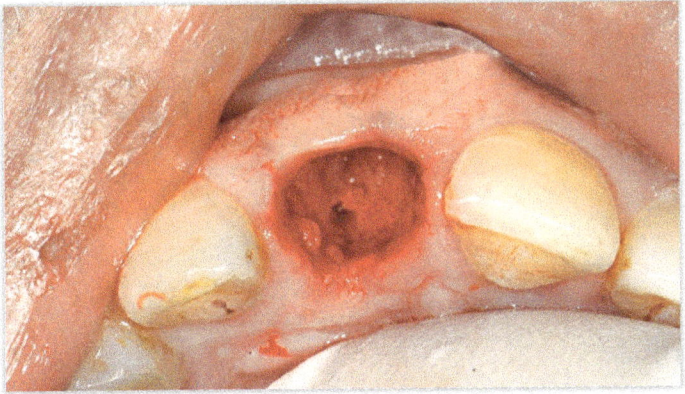

Fig. 9.6: Socket following extraction of 11. Note purchase point in apical 1/3rd of the palatal wall of the socket with precision drill.

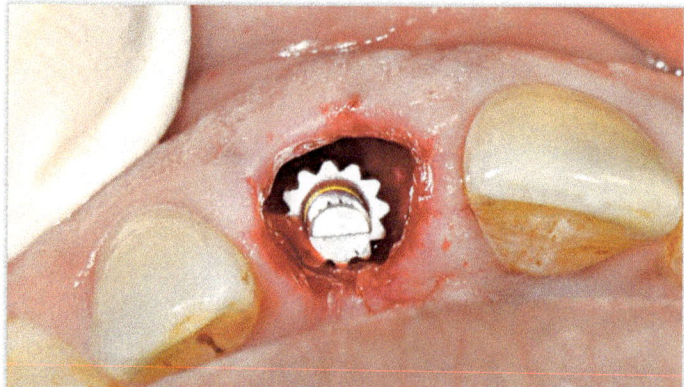

Fig. 9.7: 4.5 / 14 reamer in place 3 mm below the free gingival margin.

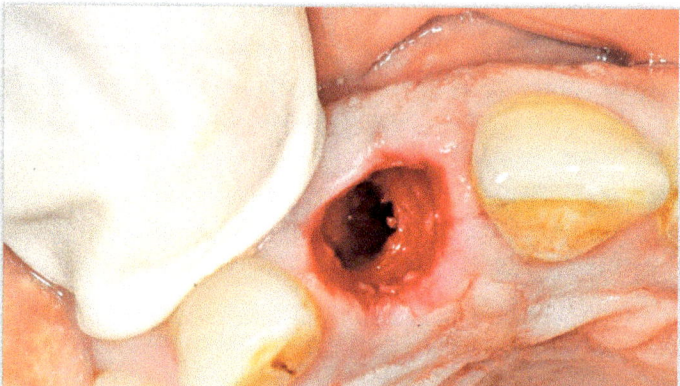

Fig. 9.8: Final osteotomy prepared towards palatal wall of socket.

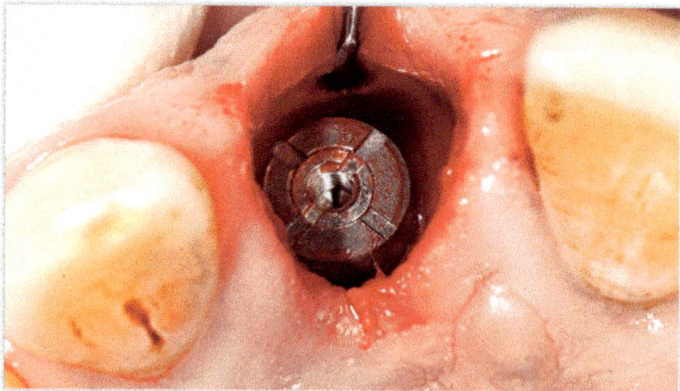

Fig. 9.9: Correct three-dimensional placement of implant.

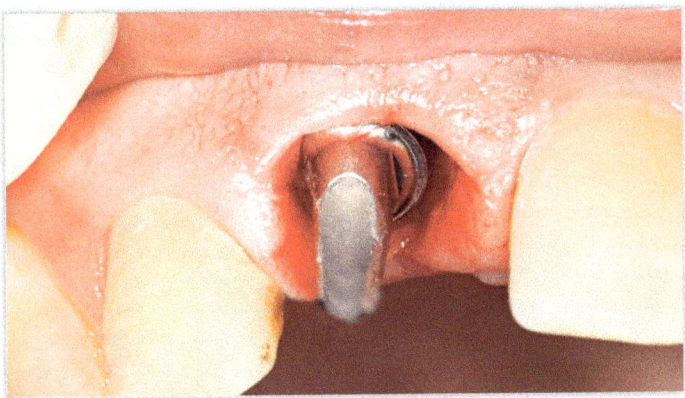

Fig. 9.10: Balance abutment 3 GH, 15° angulation.

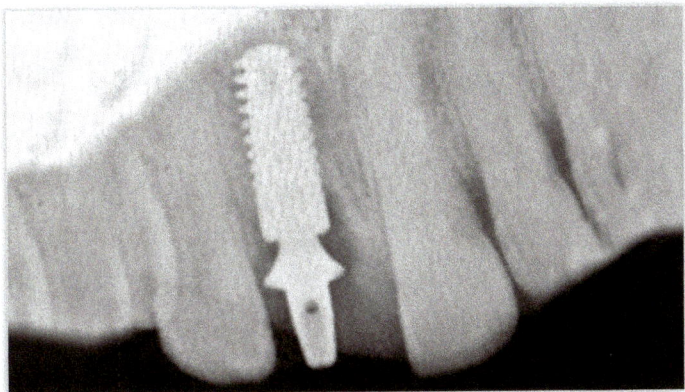

Fig. 9.11: Intra oral X-ray showing implant with abutment.

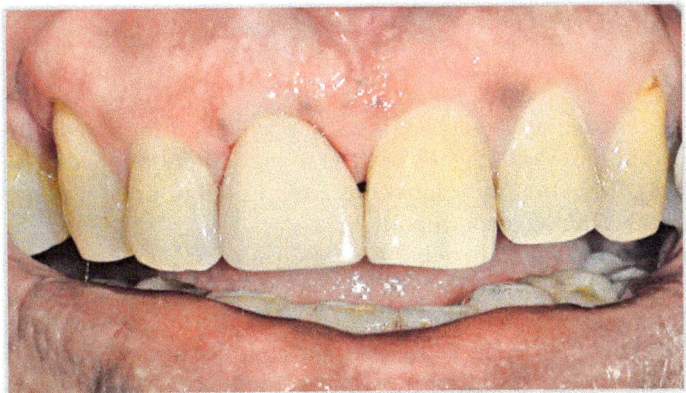

Fig. 9.12: Provisional restoration in place.

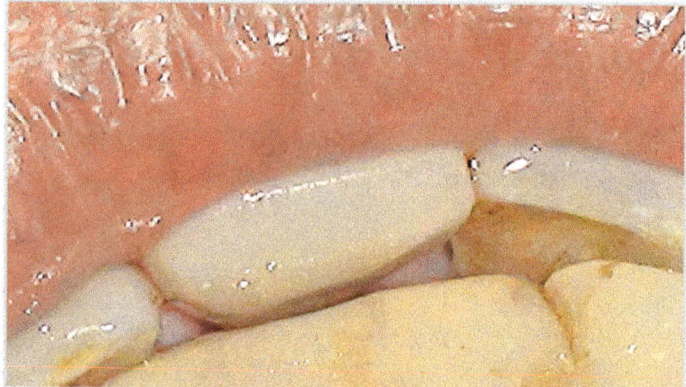

Fig. 9.13: Note the provisional restoration is kept out of occlusion.

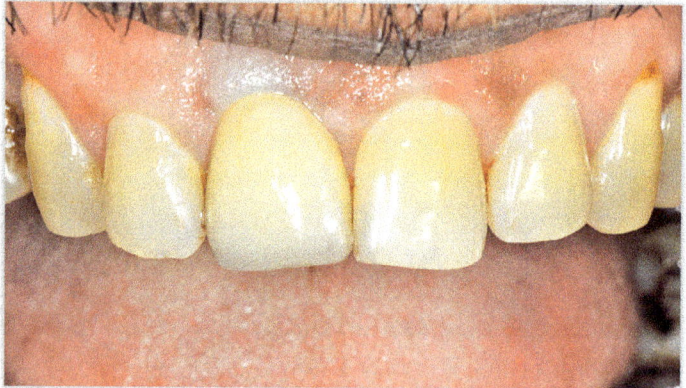

Fig. 9.14: Final restoration in place.

After supporting and sculpting the soft tissue with the provisional the final PFM restoration was delivered to the patient without removing the abutment (Fig. 9.14). The One Abutment One Time Concept preserves hard and soft tissues and is highly recommended.[4]

When the buccal plate of bone is totally absent right up to the apex of the tooth one should do a delayed approach of first grafting (GBR), wait for 6 months for bone regeneration and then place an implant to achieve optimum aesthetics (Fig. 9.15 to Fig. 9.26). The figures aptly show how a two-step staged approach gives the desired results.

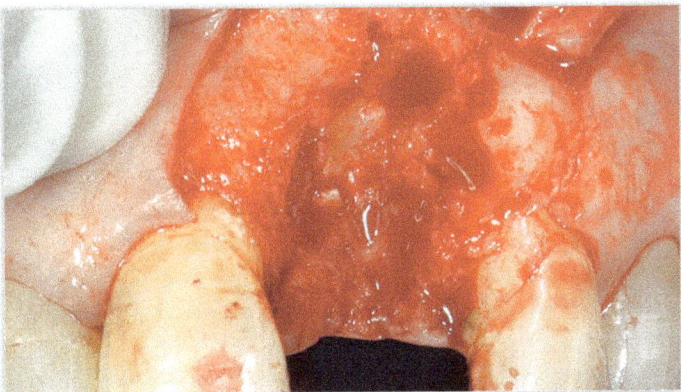

Fig. 9.15: Since there was extensive loss of buccal bone GBR is done before implant placement to achieve most predictable results.

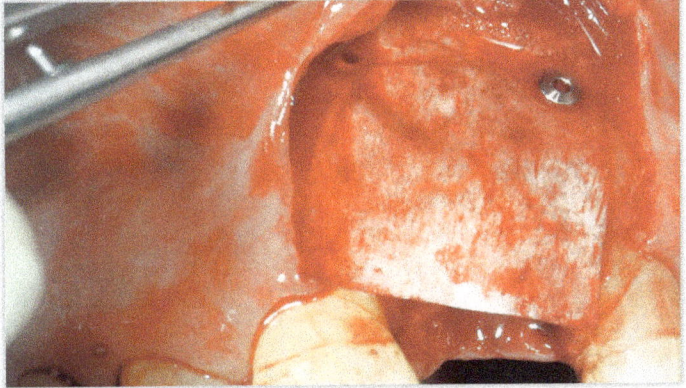

Fig. 9.16: Tacking of collagen membrane with tacking pins.

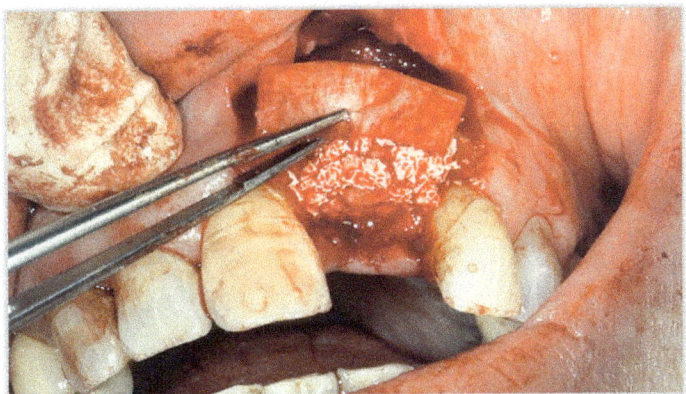

Fig. 9.17: Autogenous bone was harvested locally from the nasal spine and scrapings next to the lesion.

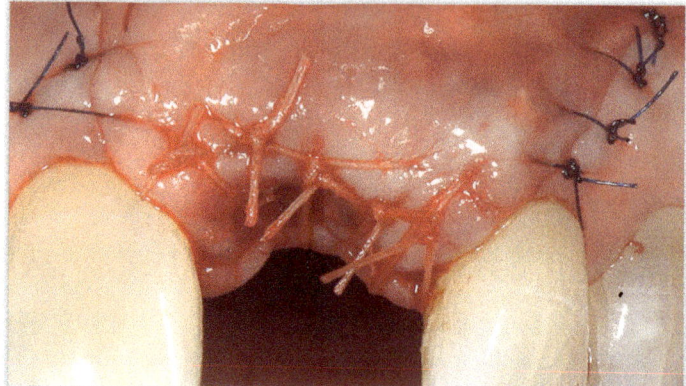

Fig. 9.18: All attempts were made to get primary closure even though there was a fresh extraction socket by splitting the flap in the apical region.

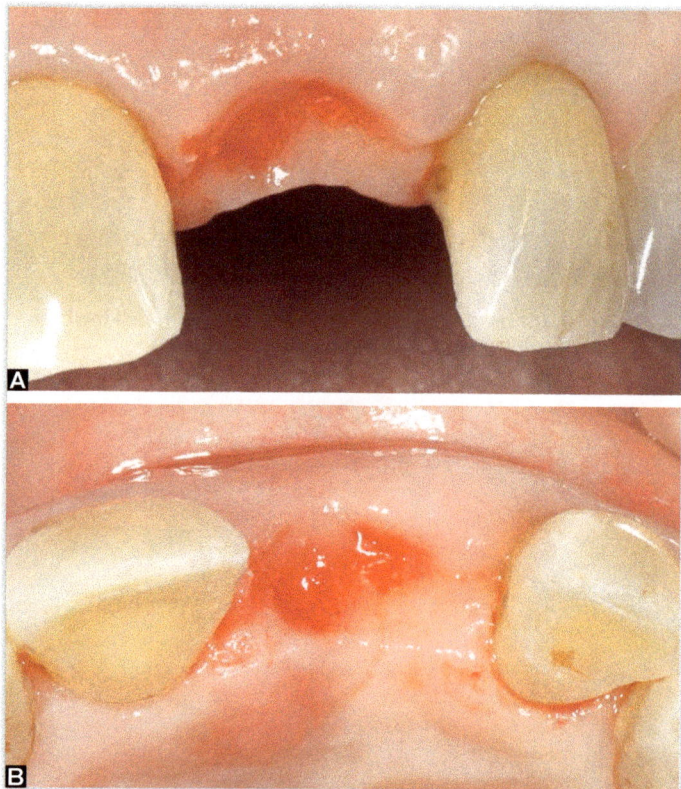

Fig. 9.19A and B: Clinical picture six months after socket grafting before flap reflection.

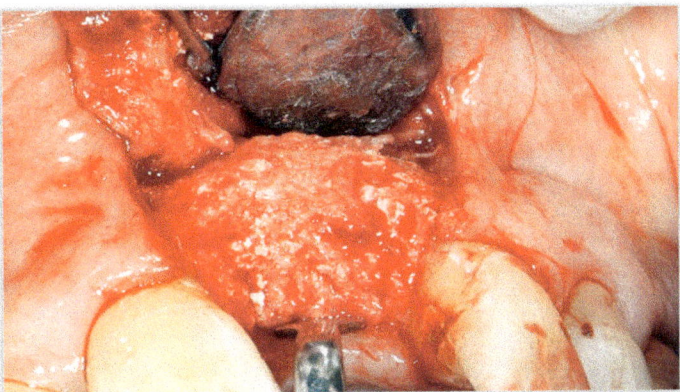

Fig. 9. 20: Note excellent regeneration of bone width resulting from GBR. Flap was reflected to remove the tacking pins.

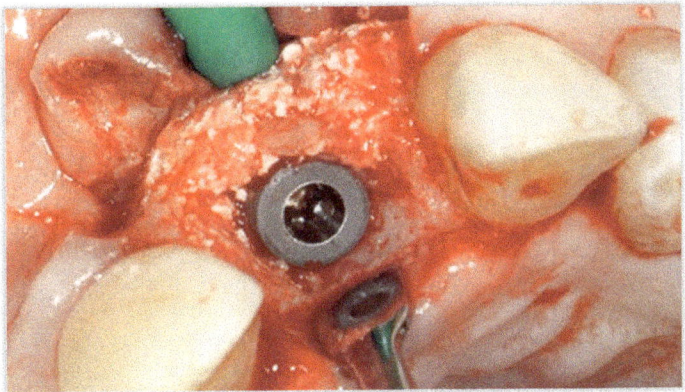

Fig. 9.21: Implant placed in correct 3D position under the incisal edge of the adjacent teeth.

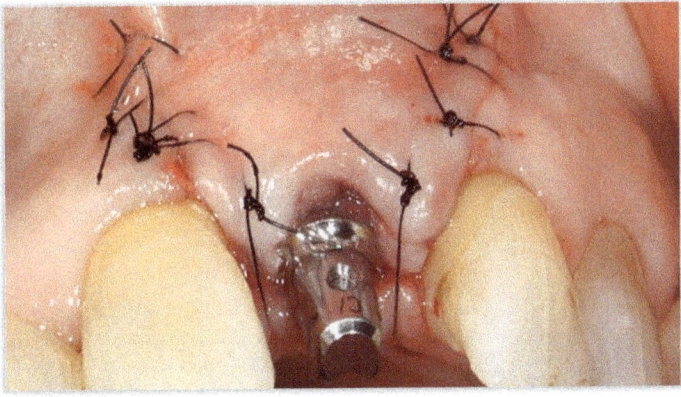

Fig. 9.22: Primary closure and abutment placed.

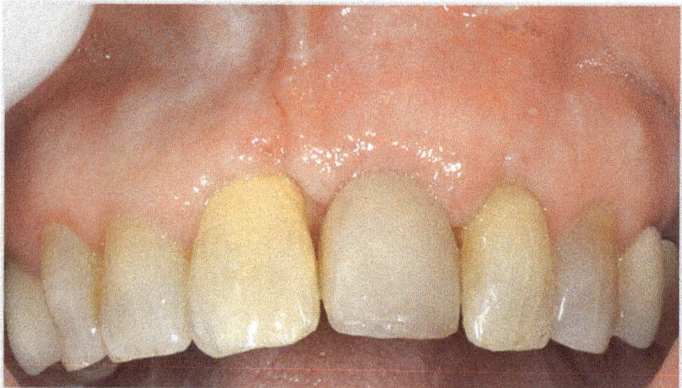

Fig. 9.23: Provisional restoration showing excellent healing after 10 days due to microsurgery.

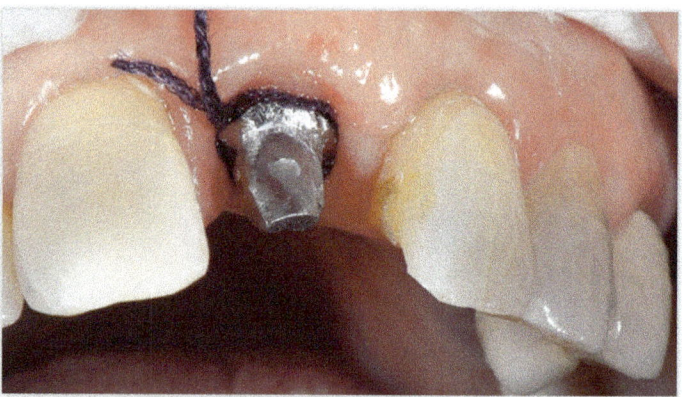

Fig. 9.24: Gingival retraction cord placed to help in removal of residual cement after cementation.

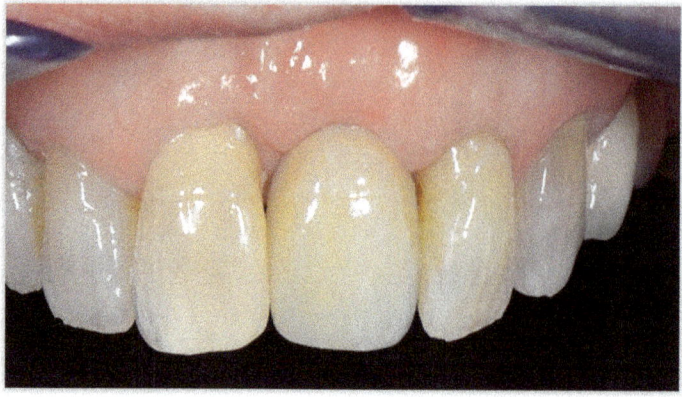

Fig. 9.25: Final crown after cenentation on day of cementation showing lack of papillae.

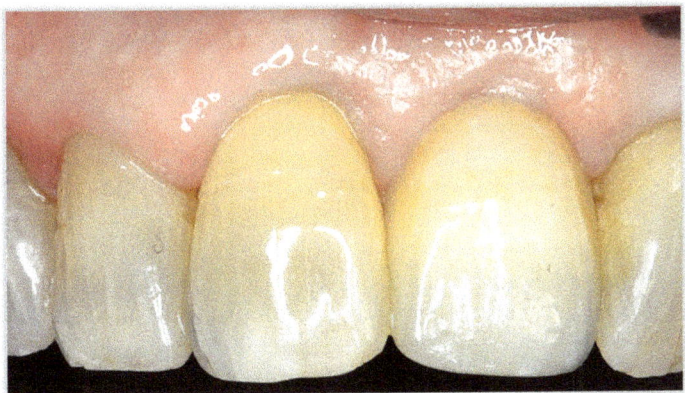

Fig. 9.26: Two-year follow-up showing spontaneous regeneration of lost papilla confirming success of GBR.

REFERENCES

1. Hermann JS, Cochran DL, Nummikoski PV, et al. Crestal bone changes around titanium implants: A radiographic evaluation of unloaded nonsubmerged and submerged implants in the canine mandible. J Periodontol. 1997;68(11):1117-30.
2. Hermann JS, Buser D, Schenk RK, et al. Crestal bone changes around titanium implants. A histometric evaluation of unloaded non-submerged and submerged implants in the canine mandible. J Periodontol. 2000;71(9):1412-24.
3. Lazzara RJ, Porter SS. Platform switching: a new concept in implant dentistry for controlling postrestorative crestal bone levels. Int J Periodontics Restorative Dent. 2006;26(1):9-17.
4. Abrahamsson I, Berglundh T, Lindhe J. The mucosal barrier following abutment dis/reconnection. An experimental study in dogs. J Clin Periodontol. 1997;24(8):569-72.

Chapter 10

The Ankylos SynCone Concept

Ledermann[1], as early as 1979 proved that immediate loading is possible with four implants placed in the mandible interforaminally and splinted with a bar. However, the bar restoration involves lengthy laboratory procedures as well as high cost. Although aesthetics and function are considered the primary object of implant therapy, patients are also seeking reduced treatment time and less cost.

The SynCone concept combines the capability of the Ankylos progressively tapered screw implants to withstand immediate loading with an innovative telescopic crown technique. It has been long proven that removable dentures can be successfully retained with telescopic crowns. However, the high cost and labor intensive laboratory procedures did not make this superior concept suitable in routine dental practice. The Ankylos SynCone system aims to combine the technical precisions with cost-effective prosthesis using prefabricated components.

It offers the option of an immediate functional overdenture chairside, while the patient is still anesthetized. The splinting of the implants which is essential for immediate loading is achieved via the prosthesis.

The conical friction locked connection between implant and abutment is particularly strong mechanically and forms a good seal. The conical connector is the basis for the success of the SynCone concept. The geometry of the cone and its high rotational stability allows angulated abutments to be aligned (made parallel) in a 360° circle, thus balancing possible axial divergencies.[2]

The Ankylos SynCone concept is also very versatile. It can be used successfully for immediate or late loading depending upon the bone quality and the primary stability of the placed implants.

IMMEDIATELY LOADED IMPLANT SUPPORTED PROSTHESIS WITH SYNCONE

Case 1

A 72-year-old lady sought treatment to improve the retention and chewing efficiency of her full lower denture (Fig. 10.1).

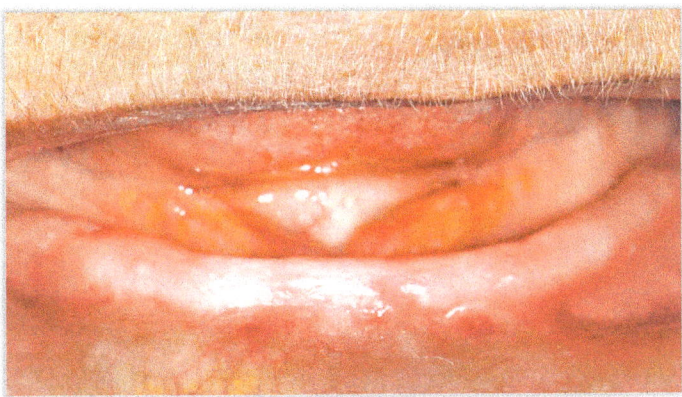

Fig. 10.1: The pre-surgical situation (note narrow ridge).

She was a non-smoker and in good health. Her existing partial upper and full lower acrylic dentures were assessed to be satisfactory in terms of extension, occlusion, and aesthetics. Further investigations by way of orthopantomograph and ridge mapping confirmed that sufficient bone was present for implant therapy. Her existing lower denture was planned to be the overdenture.

Treatment Plan

1. Placement of four interforaminal Ankylos A14 implants (3.5 mm in diameter, 14 mm in length)
2. Immediate abutment connection with Ankylos SynCone abutments
3. Immediate loading with the existing denture incorporating prefabricated telescopic copings (SynCone caps)
4. Recall and Maintenance phase.

Surgical Procedure

Under local infiltration anesthesia, a crestal incision was made leaving the median tissue bridge intact that provided a reference point of the patient's midline. This also prevents wound dehiscence secondary to frenum and muscle pull. The exposed bone was flattened and smoothened as required (Fig. 10.2). With the aid of a surgical stent (Fig. 10.3), four interforaminal sites were prepared using a 2 mm diameter pilot drill.

Direction and depth were checked with parallel gauges (Fig. 10.4).

Following the drilling protocol prescribed by the implant system, four Ankylos A14 implants were placed slightly subcrestal (Fig. 10.5). The mental nerve and its foramen should be considered always.

The cover screws are removed and prefabricated SynCone abutments with 4° taper and transgingival heights (3.0 mm) were hand torqued in (Fig. 10.6). The wound is now carefully adapted and sutured to prevent the ingress of saliva.

Prefabricated SynCone caps of gold alloy are seated on top of the SynCone abutments. Rubber dam cut collars are placed around the implants to prevent

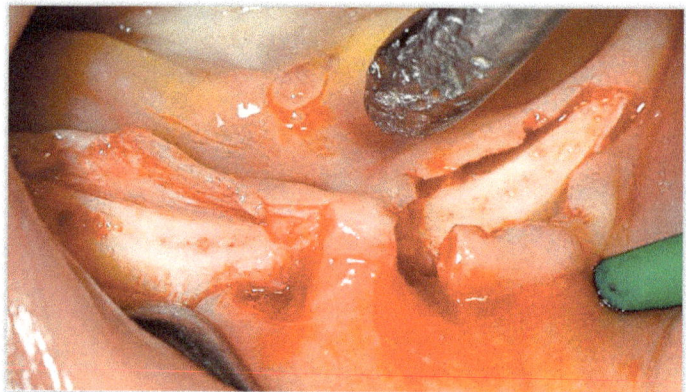

Fig. 10.2: Crestal incision with median tissue bridge intact and the sharp ridge flattened.

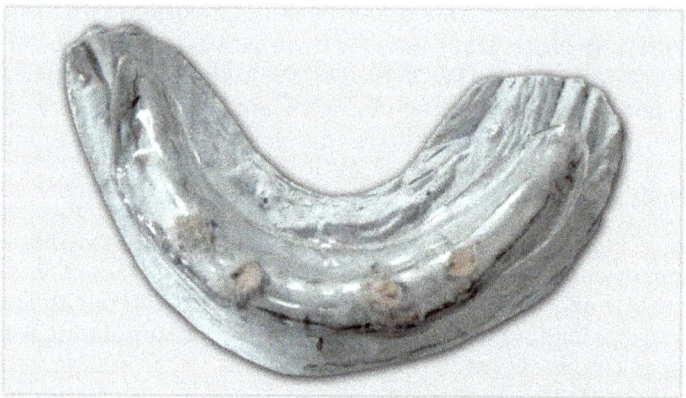

Fig. 10.3: The gutta percha markers in the radiographic stent ascertain the opening of the mental foramen with regards to the position of the implant osteotomies.

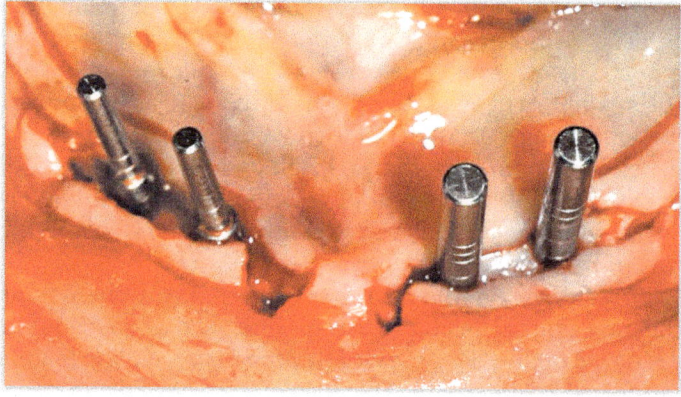

Fig. 10.4: Implant angulations checked with paralleling pins to ascertain line of draw.

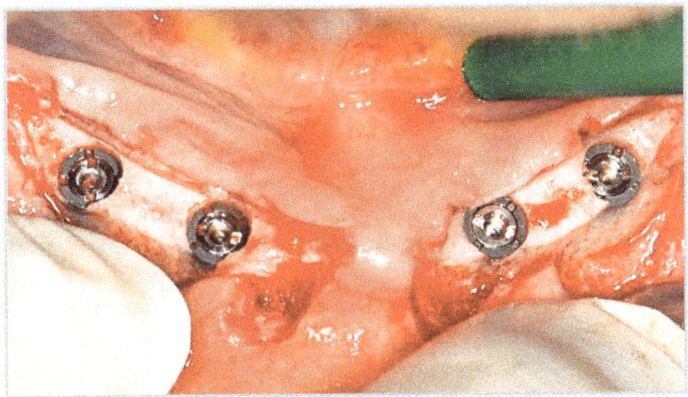

Fig. 10.5: Subcrestal placement of implants (W 3.5 L 14).

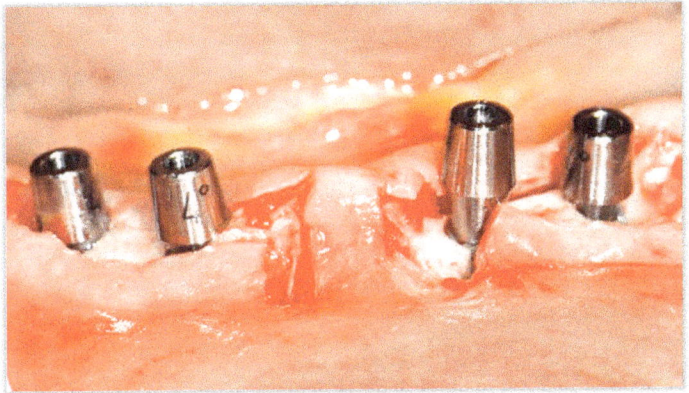

Fig. 10.6: SynCone abutments with 4° taper.

self-cure acrylic from entering the fresh wound (Fig. 10.7). Openings were created in the denture to accommodate the SynCone copings (Fig. 10.8). With the denture in place over these SynCone copings, self-cure acrylic resin in a flowing consistency is introduced into the openings in the denture and allowed to cure with the patient biting in centric relation. Once polymerization is completed, the denture is removed, finishing and polishing is then done on the modified surfaces (Fig. 10.9). The denture now with the gold caps in place is re-inserted and immediate functional loading is thus achieved.

The patient was prescribed Tresmox CV (Abbott) (amoxicillin/clavulanate potassium) 625 mg thrice daily for 5 days, Flagyl/metronidazole 400 mg thrice daily for two days, and analgesics. The patient was instructed to diligently use 0.12% Chlorhexidine Gluconate oral rinse (Periogard, Colgate India) 3 times a day for a month.

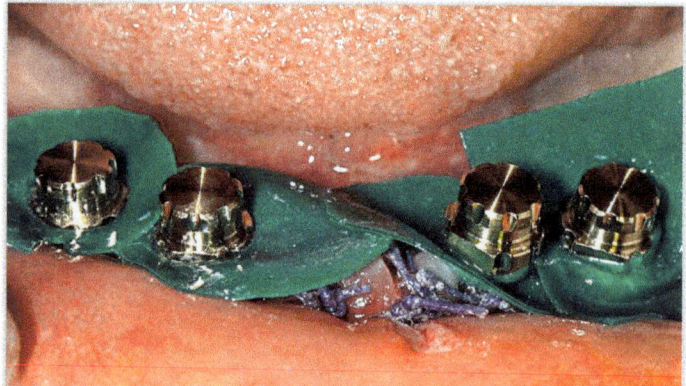

Fig. 10.7: The SynCone caps in position after suturing. Rubber dam cut-outs prevent ingress of self-polymerizing acrylic into the fresh wound.

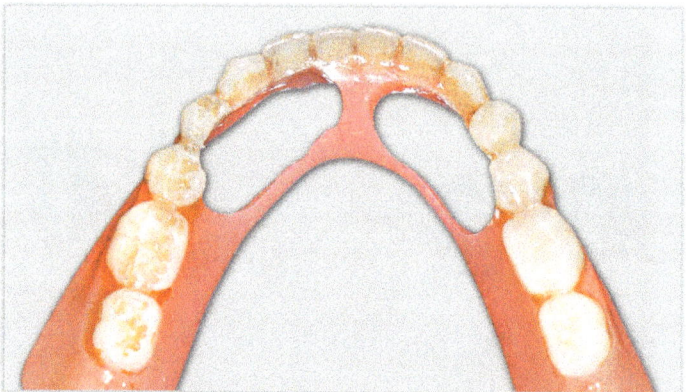

Fig. 10.8: Vent holes made in the existing denture to accommodate the SynCone housing.

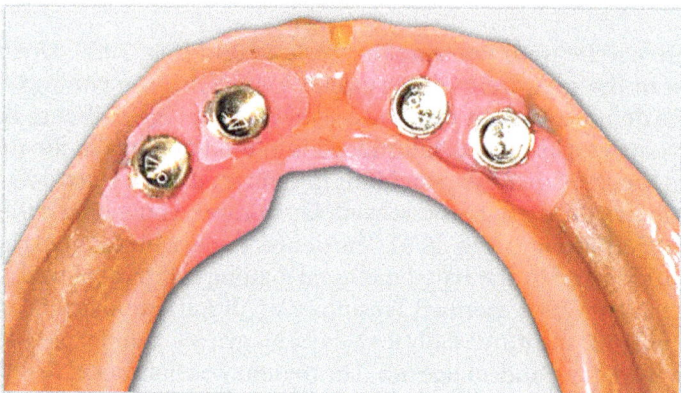

Fig. 10.9: Gold caps picked up in the existing denture after self-cure polymerization.

The patient was instructed to wear the denture continuously without removing for one week and maintain a soft diet for two weeks. After the first week the denture was removed and sutures cut. The patient was instructed to wear the denture continuously for one more week. After these two weeks the dietary restrictions were lifted and patient was taught how to maintain proper oral and denture hygiene routines. With an extra soft bristled brush (Colgate Slim and Soft Toothbrush), the patient was instructed to gently brush the mucosa and the abutments to make sure no food debris settled. The healing was monitored after one month and the gingivae had close contact with the abutments with excellent healing (Figs. 10.10 and 10.11).

Excellent Retention and Stability of Complete Maxillary Denture using SynCone Treatment Concept

Ankylos implants with only four SynCone abutments and gold caps have been well documented for long-term retention and stability of lower complete denture with only four interforaminally placed implants. However, the same

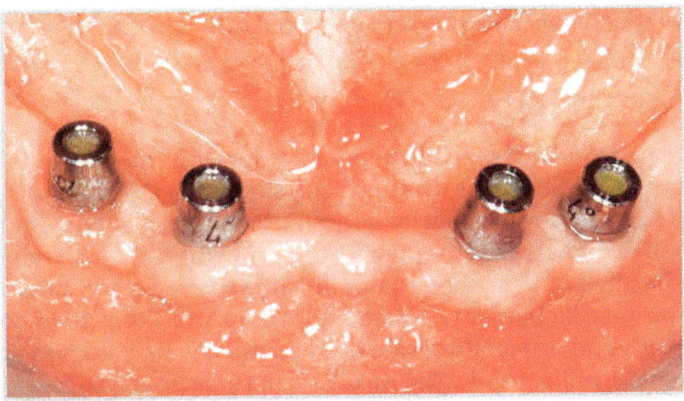

Fig. 10.10: Uneventful healing after 1 month (Note the healthy tissues).

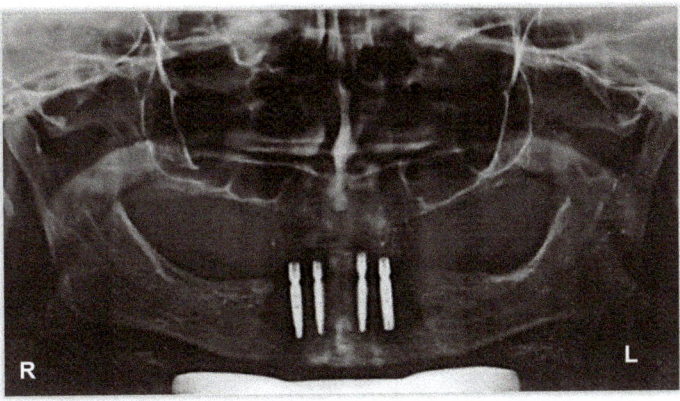

Fig. 10.11: Postoperative panoramic radiograph after 1 month.

reliability for the upper denture using SynCone is not well documented. The reason being besides the poor quality of bone of the maxilla, the greater problem in the upper jaw is getting the SynCone abutments to be parallel to each other without the assistance of the laboratory. Even after using the paralleling guide pins of the SynCone system, to get parallelism in the dental office is very difficult. Therefore, as recommended originally by Professor. Nentwig, it is safer to transfer the position of the implants by transfer impressions to the laboratory, where with the help of the parallelometer the technician can make the necessary changes in the axial inclination of the abutments using a combination of straight and angled abutments. Subsequently with the help of resin indexes, transfer the position to the patient's mouth. The case report describes how with the help of the Ankylos implant system and the technician, a difficult situation was made accurate and successful.

Case 2

Male aged 54 years desires improved retention and stability of his upper complete denture which is articulating with lower anterior natural teeth (Fig. 10.12). The patient's medical history did not exhibit any contraindications for surgery.

Treatment Planning

It was decided to stabilize his upper denture with the help of four Ankylos implants placed anterior to the maxillary sinuses since from the OPG and the CT scans, it was obvious that without sinus grafting, posterior implants were not possible. Sinus grafting was not acceptable to the patient. His upper denture was duplicated in clear acrylic and the same was used as a surgical guide to ascertain precise implant placement (Fig. 10.13). Because of poor quality bone, drills and osteotomes were used alternately to condense and prepare the osteotomy (Fig. 10.14). The Ankylos conical reamer was used finally as an osteotome with the help of an instrument especially designed by Professor Nentwig (Fig. 10.15). The bone tap was not used. Four Ankylos Implants were

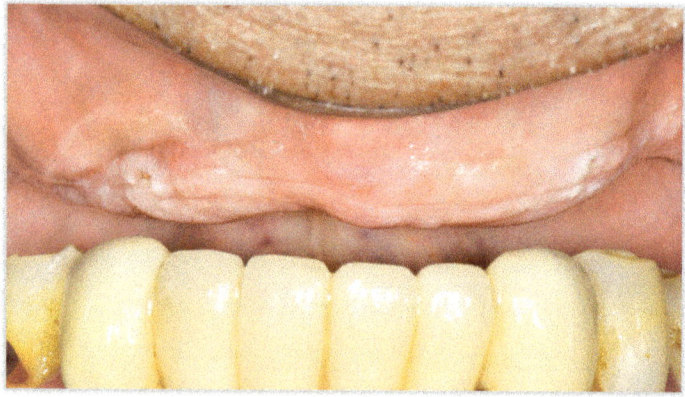

Fig. 10.12: Preoperative intraoral view.

The Ankylos SynCone Concept

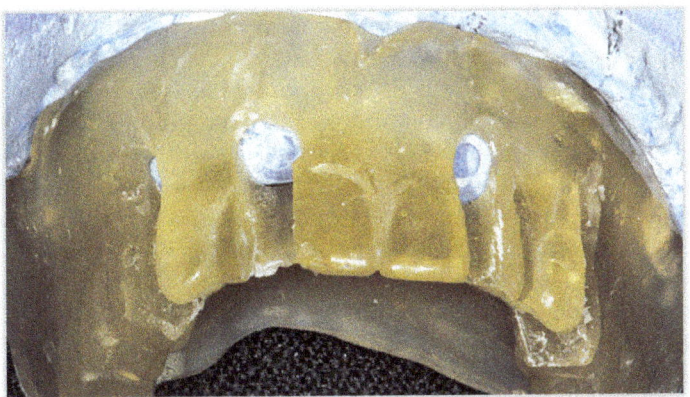

Fig. 10.13: Duplicate upper cast which will serve as surgical stent.

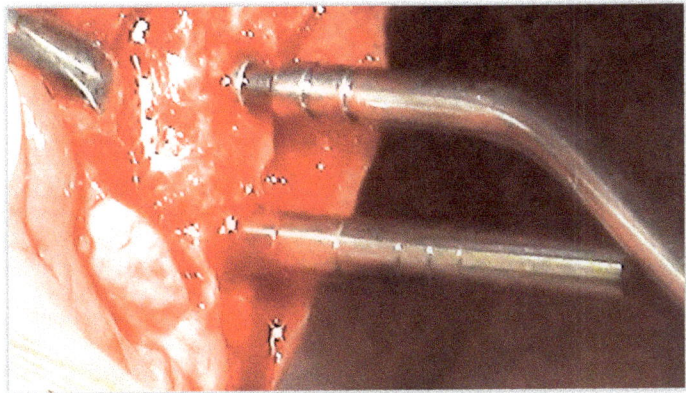

Fig. 10.14: Use of osteotome to condense bone.

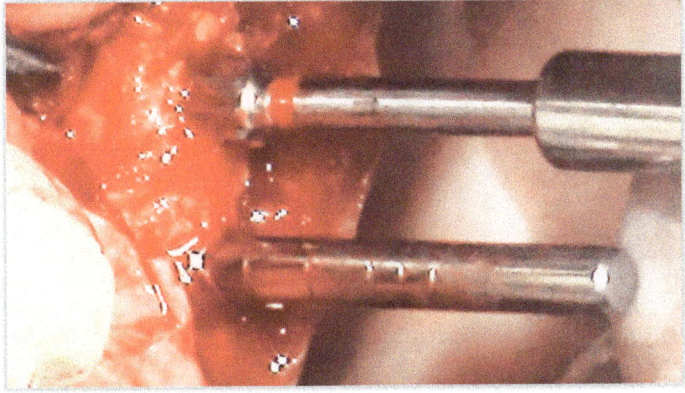

Fig. 10.15: Conical reamer used as an osteotome to condense bone. It is not rotated but malleted to the final depth of osteotome.

placed in front of the sinuses in poor quality bone, slightly subcrestally (Figs. 10.16 and 10.17). This routine of the Ankylos implant system allowed us to achieve high insertion torque even in poor quality bone. Repositioning posts were inserted into the implants after removal of the cover screws (Fig. 10.18). An impression was obtained using only light body polyvinyl siloxane material Aquasil LV (DentsplySirona) (Fig. 10.19). The putty was not used because of its rigidity. The sulcus formers were placed during the time it took for the transfer of the abutments from the laboratory to the clinic (Fig. 10.20). In the laboratory, the abutments were paralleled and the same was transferred back to the clinic with the help of resin transfer indexes (Fig. 10.21). About 6° tapered SynCone abutments were torqued in at only 15 N-cm which is the recommended torque. SynCone gold caps were placed on top of the abutments (Fig. 10.22). Punched rubber dam circular pieces were cut and placed over the

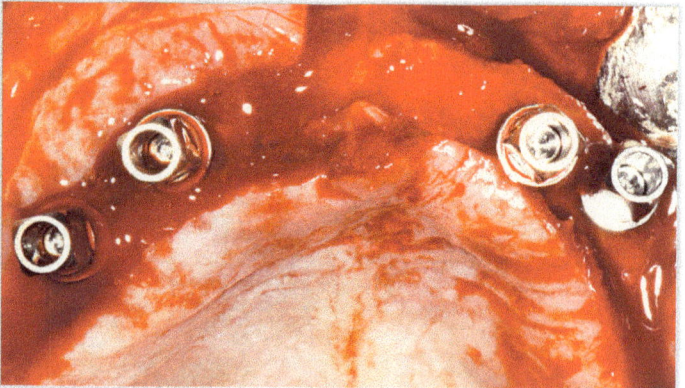

Fig. 10.16: 4 A11 Implants with their placement heads exhibiting good parallelism.

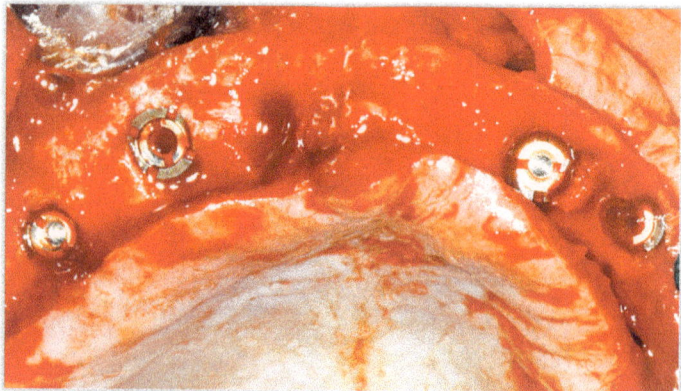

Fig. 10.17: Implants are placed 0.5 to 1 mm subcrestally.

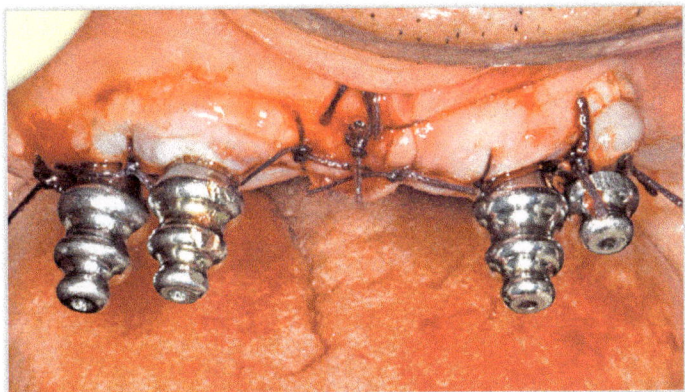

Fig. 10.18: Cover screws are removed and repositioning posts placed for closed mouth impression.

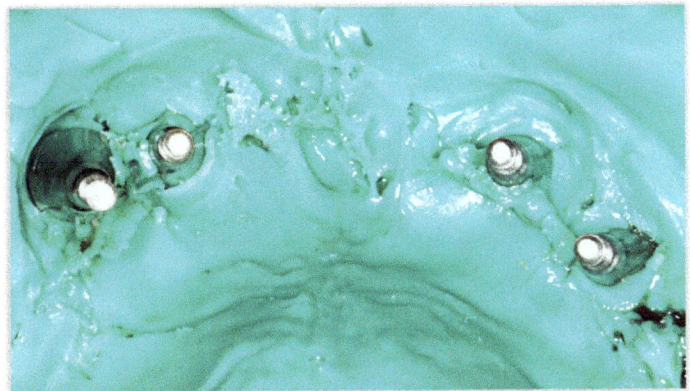

Fig. 10.19: Accurate repositioning of posts in impression before attachment to implant analogs.

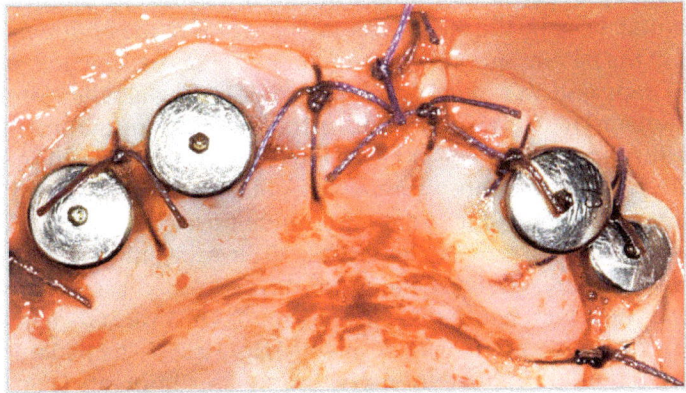

Fig. 10.20: Sulcus formers placed during the time it took to transfer abutments from laboratory.

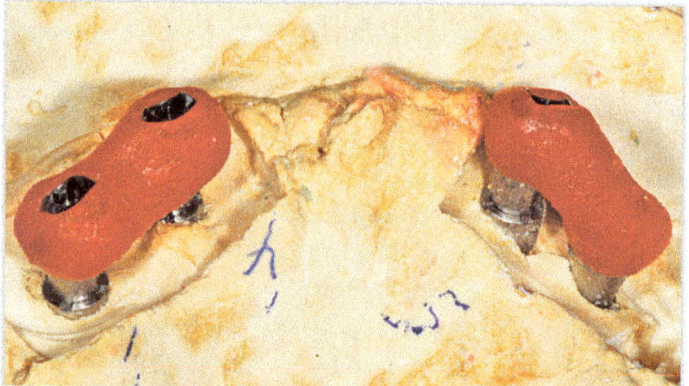

Fig. 10.21: SynCone abutments paralleled in the lab and secured with pattern resin transfer index.

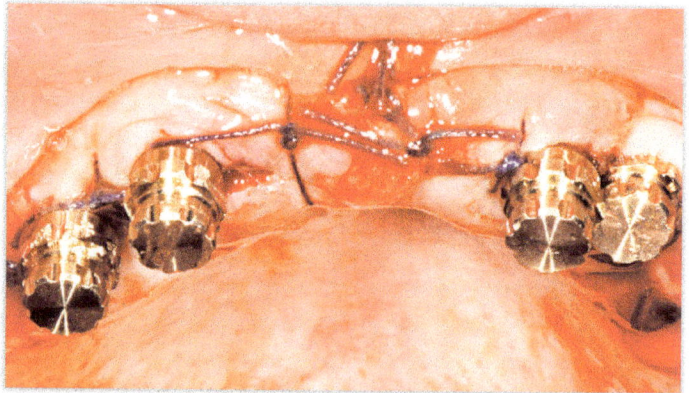

Fig. 10.22: SynCone caps in place on the abutments.

abutment to prevent the acrylic from touching the mucosa. The denture which was ground away by the technician in the region of the abutments was now placed in the patient's mouth to check for any areas which could be touching he gold caps and was suitably relieved. Self-curing acrylic resin (Lucitone Rapid Repair DentsplySirona) was mixed, placed through the openings of the denture and the patient was asked to close in centric occlusion with light pressure. Next, the denture was removed, polished and returned to the patient to wear it continuously for 15 days without removing (Fig. 10.23). The patient was instructed to eat only soft food. After 15 days the patient returned and the sutures were removed. The patient was dismissed and asked to return again after one week for a check-up (Fig. 10.24). An OPG was taken after 3 weeks showing good placement of the implants (Fig. 10.25). The patient was happy with the retention of his denture with only four implants (Fig. 10.26). He has been asked to return after 6 months when we plan to make a new upper denture with cast framework to further improve the stability and strength of

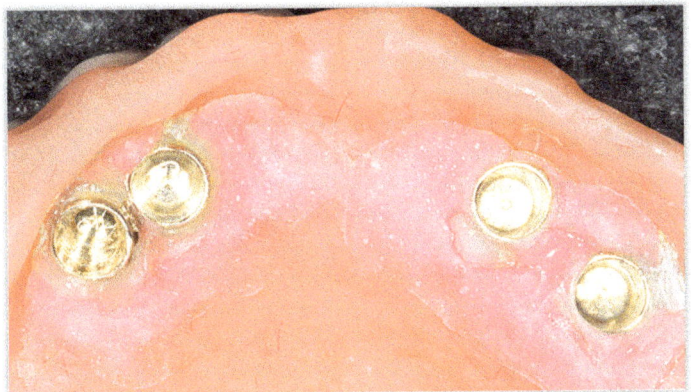

Fig. 10.23: SynCone caps picked up in upper complete denture.

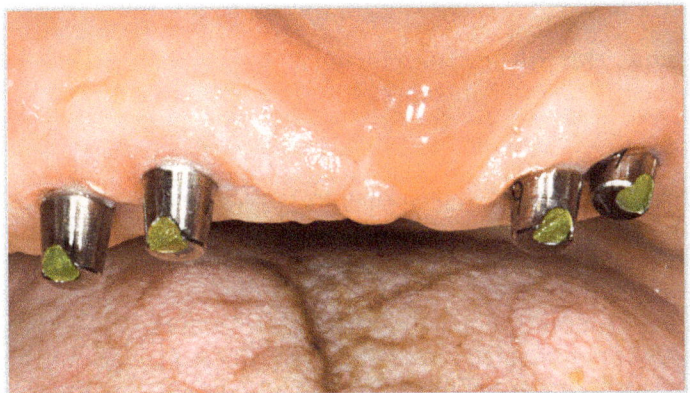

Fig. 10.24: Healing after 3 weeks.

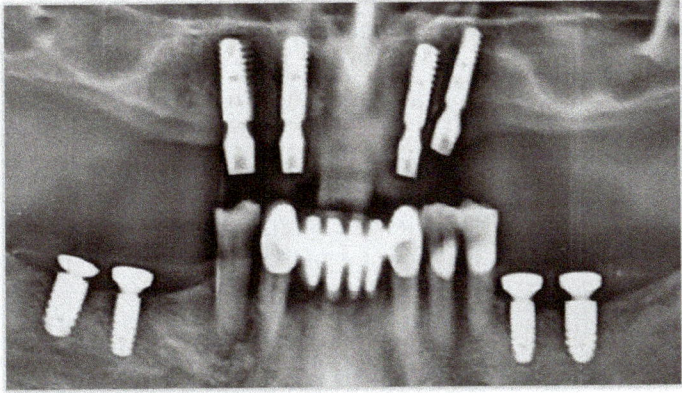

Fig. 10.25: OPG after placement of implants in upper and lower jaw.

146 Clinical Guide to Oral Implantology: Step by Step Procedures

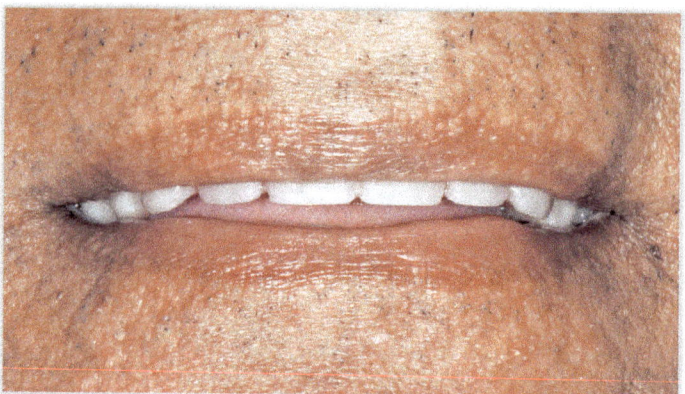

Fig. 10.26: Smile after rehabilitation with complete denture supported by four ankylos implants.

the denture. This will be done after rehabilitation of his lower posterior teeth with implant supported prosthesis.

Conclusion

Retention of the upper complete denture is usually not a problem as compared to the lower denture. However, in cases where the lower natural teeth exist especially only anteriors as in the above case, retention and stability suffers. Also without implants the bone in the upper edentulous jaw underneath complete dentures is rapidly resorbed due to considerable forces generated by the lower natural teeth. In such circumstances placing only four Ankylos implants with SynCone abutments and gold caps achieves excellent stability, retention and also prevents resorption of the edentulous ridge. This can be achieved in a fast economical way with the assistance of the laboratory. In the above case, the palatal portion of the denture was not removed, since it adds strength and stability to the acrylic denture. However, once the denture is strengthened with metal casting after a period of 6 months, the palate will no longer be needed.

Delayed Loading of Implants Using the SynCone Concept in Compromised Situation

Although the SynCone concept was developed for immediate functional loading, it is extremely versatile and can be used with submerged implants and delayed loading where the bone quality is not good and primary stability is inadequate.

Case 3

Male-aged 75 years is not happy with retention and stability of his upper denture which is in articulation with lower natural teeth.

Diagnosis and Treatment Planning

The patient requested minimum surgical procedures and declined sinus grafting. Looking at the advanced age of the patient, it was decided to treat him with implant supported removable denture using the SynCone concept. Four Ankylos implants A11 were planned to be placed in front of the pneumatised sinus cavity.

Intraoperative Procedures

Crestal incision slightly palatally was placed with two posterior releasing incisions (Fig. 10.27). On exposure of the ridge, it was noticed that the ridge quality and volume was very poor. All attempts were made to drill at the expense of the palatal cortical plate. Also after the initial pilot drill osteotomes were used instead of drills to condense the trabeculae of bone to improve density (Fig. 10.28). Four implants were placed with limited primary stability, especially the upper right implant in the canine region had poor primary stability and the buccal bone had a green stick fracture (Fig. 10.29). Allogenic bone (Rocky Mountain, USA) was placed bucally to add stability to the buccal plate in the right canine region. The bone substitute was covered with a collagen membrane (Bio-Gide, Geistlich, Switzerland) (Fig. 10.30). The wound edges were closed with interrupted sutures.

Second Stage Surgery

After a healing period of 4 months at the time of second stage surgery, it was noticed that the right implant in the grafted canine region was mobile and was therefore removed. It was therefore decided to use only three implants with the SynCone concept (Fig. 10.31). After placing sulcus formers and waiting for a period of 10 days, impression procedures were started using the open tray technique and a custom-made acrylic

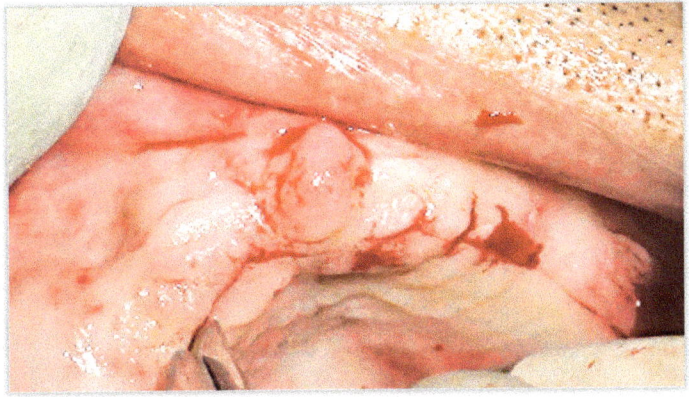

Fig. 10.27: Initial incision placed slightly palatally.

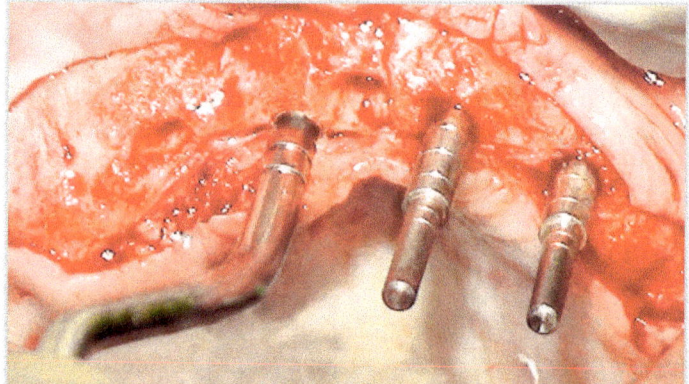

Fig. 10.28: Osteotome used to condense the bone.

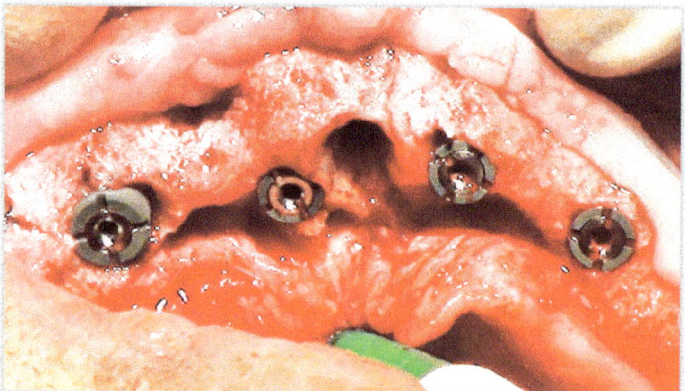

Fig. 10.29: Note the green-stick fracture in area of upper right canine.

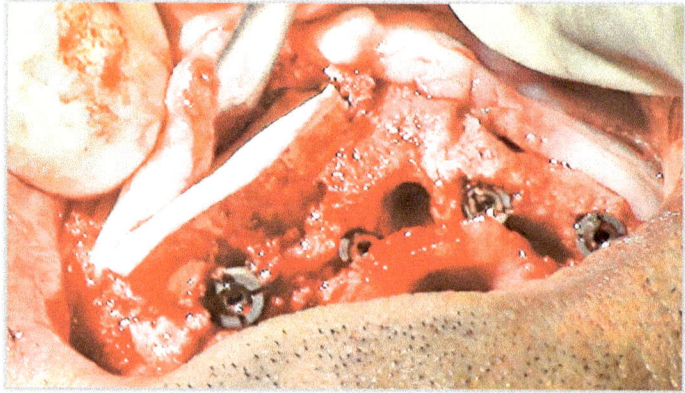

Fig. 10.30: GBR performed to support green-stick fracture.

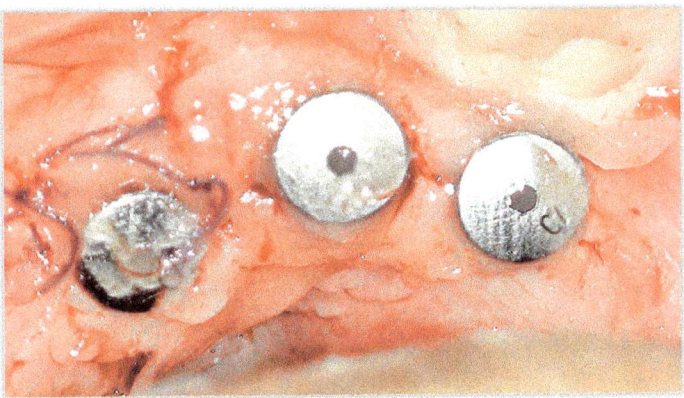

Fig. 10.31: Sulcus formers placed after 2nd stage surgery.

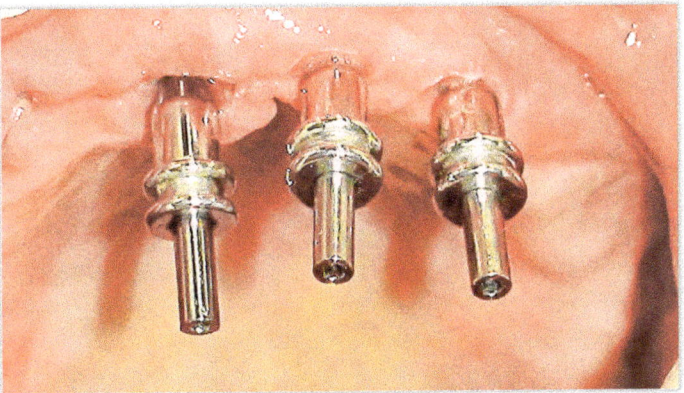

Fig. 10.32: Open tray impression posts in place.

tray (Fig. 10.32). The impression posts were picked up in the impression and the position of the abutments were transferred to the laboratory to make a metal denture framework (Fig. 10.33). With the help of accurate and sturdy resin transfer indexes the SynCone abutments paralleled by the laboratory were transferred to the patients mouth and torqued in at 15 N-cm (Fig. 10.34) (During the interim period when the castings were incorporated in the new denture, the patient's old denture was relieved in the area of the abutments and relined with a soft denture liner (Fig. 10.35). The gold caps were placed on the abutments and the metal casting was tried in. A dual-cured resin cement Calibra (DentsplySirona) was used to lute the gold coping intraorally to the metal framework (Fig. 10.36). The framework and gold caps position was transferred to the laboratory with

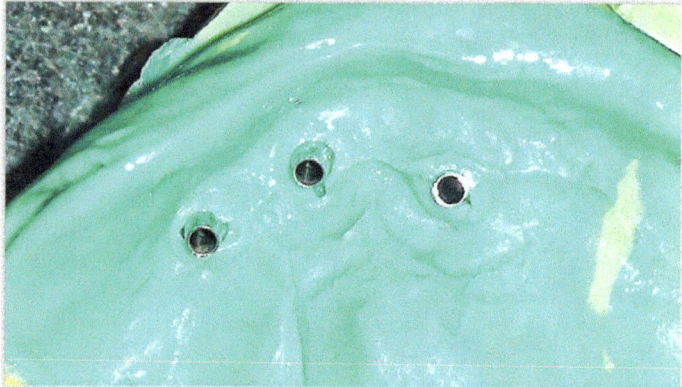

Fig. 10.33: Pick-up impression with the posts.

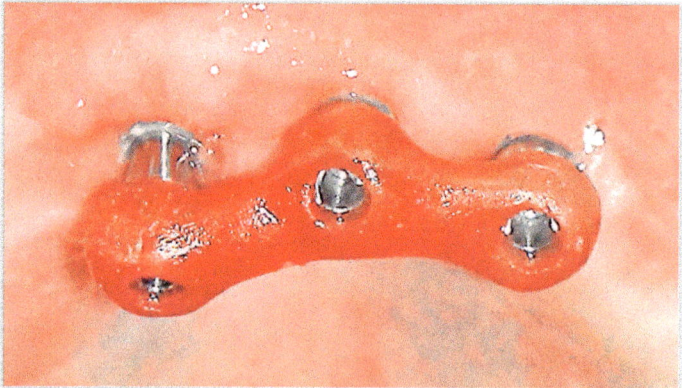

Fig. 10.34: Accurate transfer of abutment position from lab to patient's mouth.

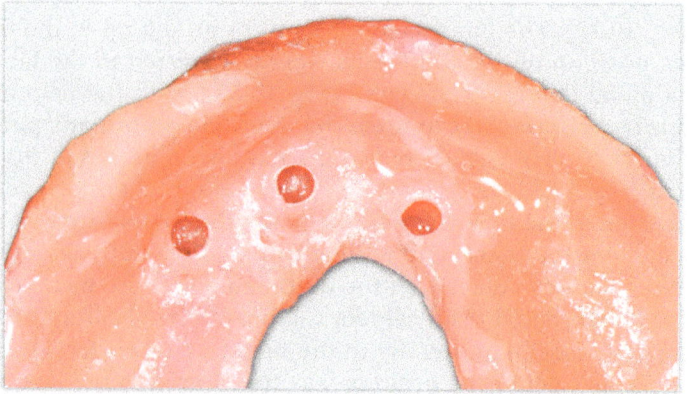

Fig. 10.35: Soft denture liner during interim period.

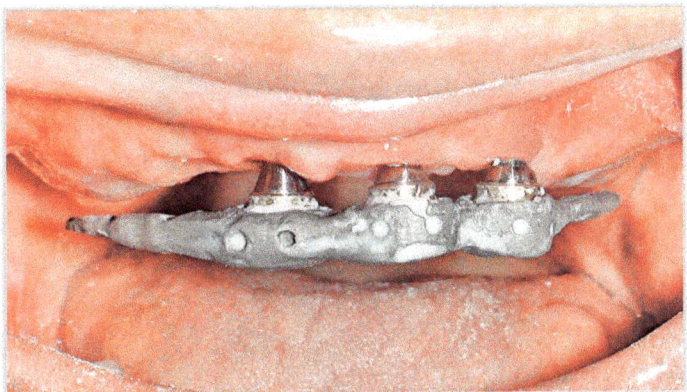

Fig. 10.36: SynCone gold caps cemented to the metal framework.

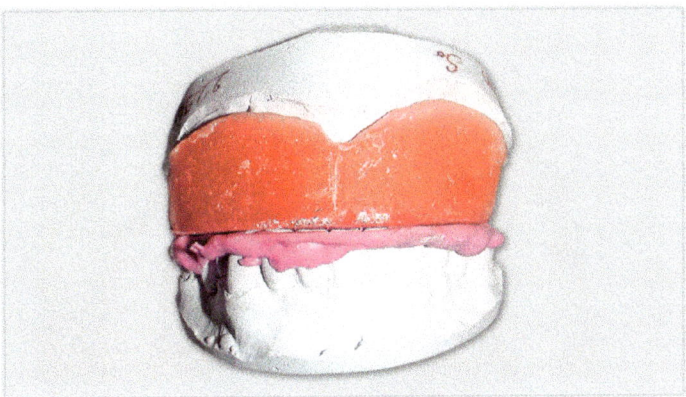

Fig. 10.37: Jaw relation recorded.

the help of an impression in polyvinyl silicone (Aquasil LV DentsplySirona). The laboratory constructed a self-cure base plate with wax rims. The same was used to record the jaw relations (Fig. 10.37). A face bow transfer was also done. After the setting trial was confirmed with regards to correct centric relation, aesthetics and phonetics, the laboratory completed the upper removable prosthesis incorporating the casting and the gold caps (Figs. 10.38 and 10.39). As per the patients wish the denture was made without covering the palate. However, even without the palate and only with three abutments, there was excellent retention and stability (Fig. 10.40). The patient has been followed up since the last eight years with no complications and he is able to masticate all types of food. Although his hygiene is far from ideal, no signs of peri-implantitis are evident to date (Fig. 10.41).

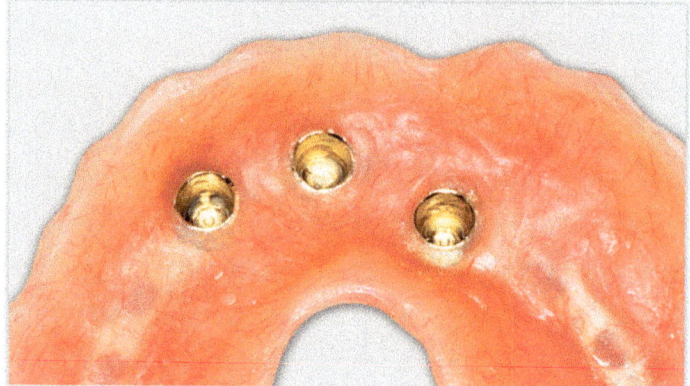

Fig. 10.38: Intaglio surface of denture.

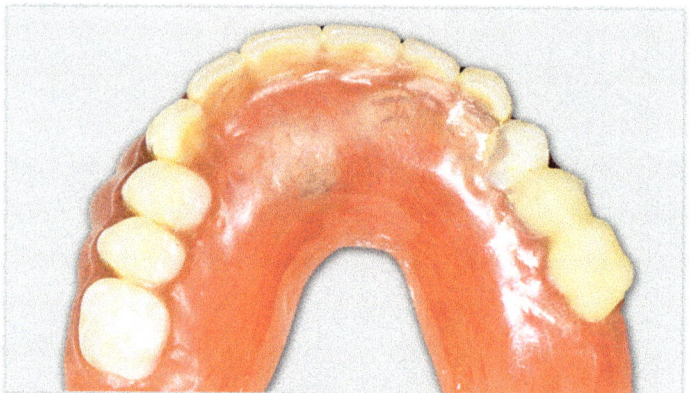

Fig. 10.39: Polished surface of denture.

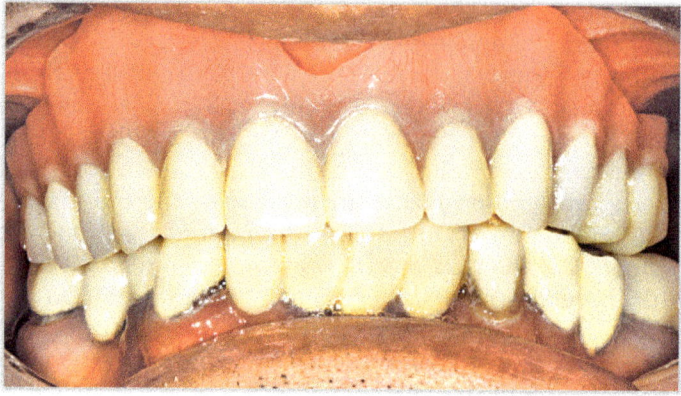

Fig. 10.40: Denture in patients mouth in centric occlusion.

The Ankylos SynCone Concept

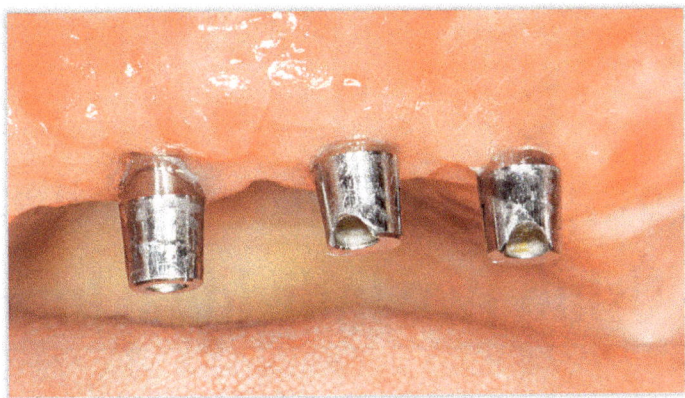

Fig. 10.41: Good maintenance of hard and soft tissues after 1 year.

REFERENCES

1. Ledermann P. Bar-prosthetic management of the edentulous mandible by means of plasma-coated implantation with titanium screws. Dtsch Zahnarztl Z.1979; 34(12):907-11.
2. Chmeielewski K. Practice success with SynCone. Identity 2008; 1:24-7.

Chapter 11

Complete Denture Stabilization Using Two Individual Implants

The Ankylos Snap Attachment is an economical method of stabilizing mucosa supported removable prosthesis. It is particularly suited in elderly patients to stabilize their complete dentures, thus vastly improving their quality of life. The Snap Attachments are resilient, permit rotational and transitional movements, although they stabilize the mucosa supported denture. Abutments of the Snap Attachment consist of a primary element which is screwed into the implant and a secondary component which has to be fixed into the denture.

The Snap Attachment abutments are placed on two implants that have been inserted in the interforaminal region preferably in the region of the canines. Since the attachment are single units and not splinted to each other with a bar, it has several advantages as under:
- It is easier for the patient to clean and is therefore more hygienic
- It requires less space and therefore is ideally suited where interarch distance is limited.
- It is more comfortable for patients since tongue space is maximized due to less area occupied by the attachment.[1,2]

However as with all hybrid dentures (mucosa and implant supported) regular recall and maintenance is required. The recall intervals should be shorter compared to a solely implant supported overdenture since the hybrid denture always requires relining due to resorption of the posterior ridges where it is mucosa supported. If periodic relining is not done there is a danger of overloading of the implant abutments.

The Snap Attachment consists of a male part which is spherical in shape and a female part which remains in the denture. The male part is made of titanium and the female part is made of precious alloy to prevent abrasive wear.

Adjustment of the friction between the male and female parts can be done with activating- deactivating instrument.

The Snap Attachments are screwed into the implant using the ratchet insert and prosthetic ratchet. The abutments are screwed into the implants at 25 Ncm.

The attachment females are fixed into the denture directly in the mouth using self cure acrylic resin. For this purpose, the female is placed on the abutment with the enclose silicone sleeve. With its lower end the enclosed silicone seizes the hexagon of the snap attachment abutment and with its upper end it encloses the lamellae of the female. Thus, the silicone sleeve holds the

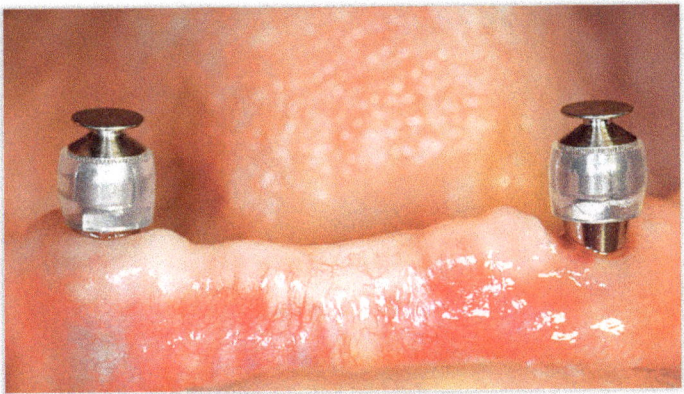

Fig. 11.1: Silicone sleeve covering the lamella as well as the hex of the abutment.

female in the axial direction of the abutment. Note it is very important that the silicone sleeve is in place on the male and the female parts during the pick-up of the female part in the denture by self cure resin (Fig. 11.1). Also ensure that no acrylic resin reaches between the lamellae of the female part. Remove the silicone sleeve after the polymerization is complete.

CASE REPORT

Female aged 85 years reports with loss of fixed partial denture replacing 31, 32, 33, 34, 41, 42, 43, 44 (Fig. 11.2).

She requests replacement of the same for function and esthetics in an economic way. It was decided to extract the remaining roots and place 2 implants immediately, wait for 3 months for osseointegration and rehabilitate her with a complete denture stabilized with snap attachments on the implants. Subsequently after 3 months lower complete denture was prepared with the sulcus formers in place (Fig. 11.3). After completion of the denture the sulcus formers were removed and Ankylos snap abutments were torqued in at 25Ncm. Gold snap attachments were placed on top of the spherical abutments and the same was covered with silicone sleeve. Care was taken to see that the silicone sleeve covered the lamellae of the female gold cap as also they reached up to the hex of the abutment (see Fig. 11.1). The denture was relieved in the place of the abutments and placed in the mouth to see that there was enough clearance all around (Fig. 11.4). Cold cure acrylic was poured into the holes to pick-up the female attachment. The patient was asked to gently close in centric occlusion and to keep this position for 5 minutes for complete curing of the acrylic resin. Subsequently the denture was removed with the picked up gold female attachment. The silicone sleeve was removed (Figs. 11.5A and B). The denture was replaced back. The patient was satisfied with the retention and stability of the lower denture. The patient was instructed in the hygiene of the abutments and the denture. The patient was placed on a soft diet for the first two weeks. She was also strictly instructed to rinse twice daily with a 0.12 % Chlorhexidine (Periogard, Colgate Oral Care, Mumbai, India)

156 Clinical Guide to Oral Implantology: Step by Step Procedures

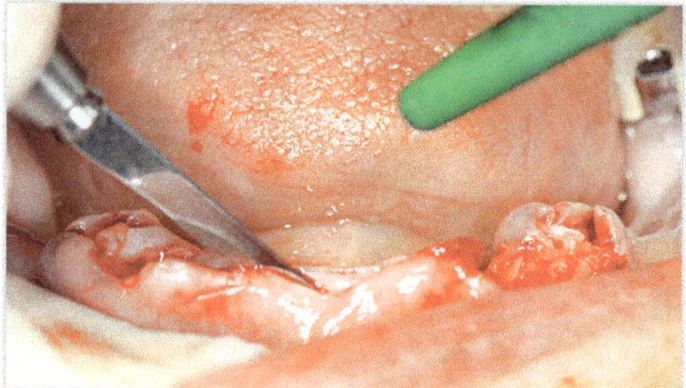

Fig. 11.2: Intraoral picture after failure of fixed partial dentures.

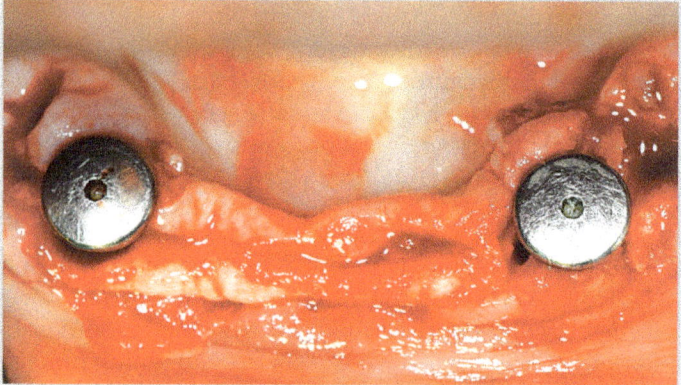

Fig. 11.3: Sulcus formers in place.

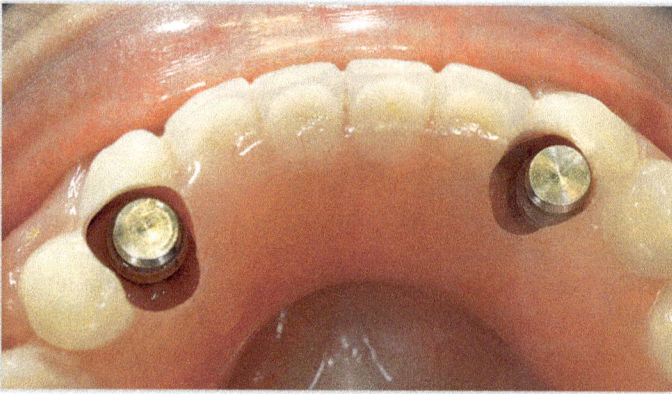

Fig. 11.4: Denture relieved in the region of the snap attachments.

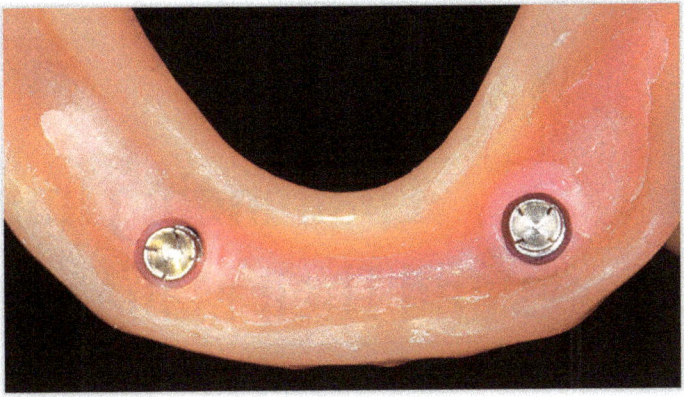

Fig. 11.5A: Intaglio surface of the denture after removal of the silicone sleeves.

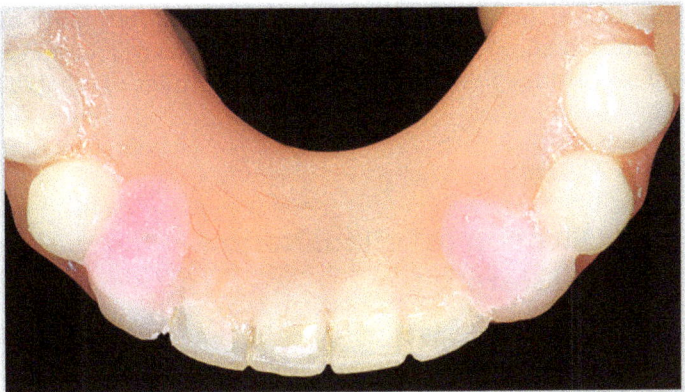

Fig. 11.5B: Final polished surface of the denture.

CONCLUSION

Two interforaminal implant supported overdenture has been shown to improve the quality of life of lower complete denture wearers.[3]

REFERENCES

1. Attard NJ, David LA, Zarb GA. Immediate loading of implants with mandibular overdentures: one-year clinical results of a prospective study. Int J Prosthodont. 2005;18(6):463-70.
2. Chiapasco M, Gatti C, Rossi E, Haefliger W, Markwalder TH. Implant-retained mandibular overdentures with immediate loading. A retrospective multicenter study on 226 consecutive cases. Clin Oral Implants Res. 1997;8(1):48-57.
3. Feine JS, Carlsson GE, Awad MA, Chehade A, Duncan WJ, Gizani S, et al. The McGill consensus statement on overdentures. Mandibular two-implant overdentures as first choice standard of care for edentulous patients. Montreal, Quebec. Int J Oral Maxillofac Implants. 2002;17(4):601-2.

Chapter 12

Challenging Implant Cases and Their Management

Today implantologists are ever pushing the envelope further and from their studies we have come to know that in selected cases and by using the proper materials and techniques it is possible to rehabilitate patients quickly, comfortably, esthetically and functionally. This series will present cases which will challenge some of the old and current principles of rehabilitation with implants.

CASE 1

Challenge: Economic Rehabilitation with Fixed Restoration

Male aged 73 years is brought to the clinic by his daughters who wish that his mouth be rehabilitated so that he may be able to masticate his food. They also expressed a desire for an economic plan of treatment. On asking for his chief complaint the patient reports difficulty in masticating his food. On examination, i.e. clinical and radiographic it is observed that most of his teeth are diseased and will require extractions (Fig. 12.1).

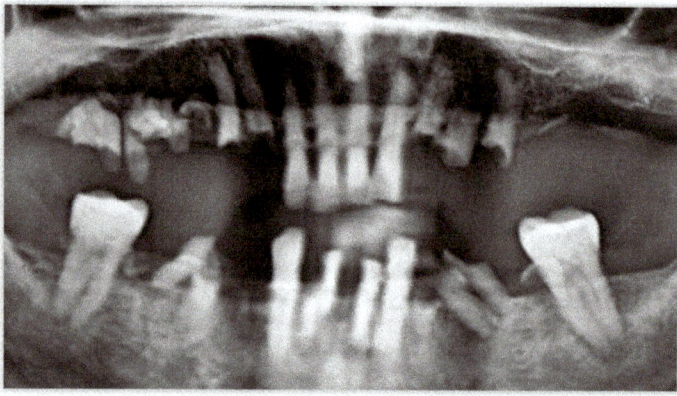

Fig. 12.1: Preoperative OPG showing neglect and diseased condition of the dentition.

TREATMENT PLAN

Keeping in mind the need for cost effective treatment it was decided to preserve four upper incisors 11, 12, 21 and 22. In the lower the two canines and two second molars would be preserved after endodontic treatment. The lower rehabilitation would be a tooth and implant splinted fixed prosthesis with only two implants placed between the canines and the second molars. The upper rehabilitation would be with a cast partial denture.

TREATMENT

All nonsalvageable teeth were extracted and after waiting for a healing period of about 2 months' implants were placed in the region between the second molar and the first molar. After waiting for a further period of two months for osseointegration repositioning posts were placed and a crown and bridge impression of the prepared teeth and the repositioning posts was taken using Aquasil Putty and Aquasil LV (Dentsply Sirona) (Figs. 12.2 and 12.3). Interocclusal registrations using a face bow were taken (Fig. 12.4). A ceramo-metal fixed restoration was made in 2 parts splinting the natural second molar, implant and canine with cantilevers of lateral and central incisors (Fig. 12.5A).

DISCUSSION

The case report exemplifies that it is possible to rehabilitate aged persons successfully with minimal implants and by preserving the natural salvageable teeth. It is the authors' opinion that wherever natural teeth can be salvaged they can be joined to implants especially those implants which have a strong conical implant abutment connection.[1] Since lower complete dentures are more difficult for patients to manage, it was decided to do a fixed prosthesis in the lower jaw and a removable cast partial denture in the upper jaw.

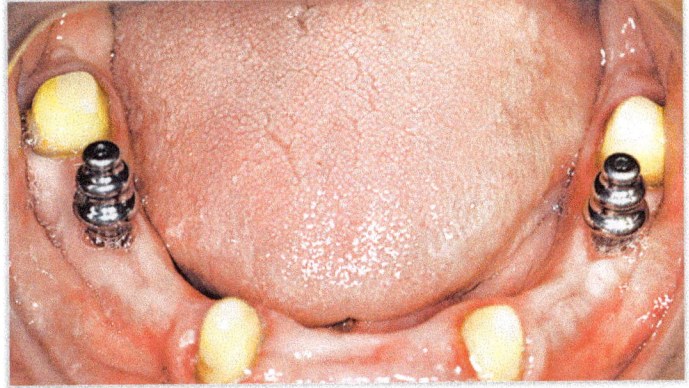

Fig. 12.2: Intraoral view with repositioning posts.

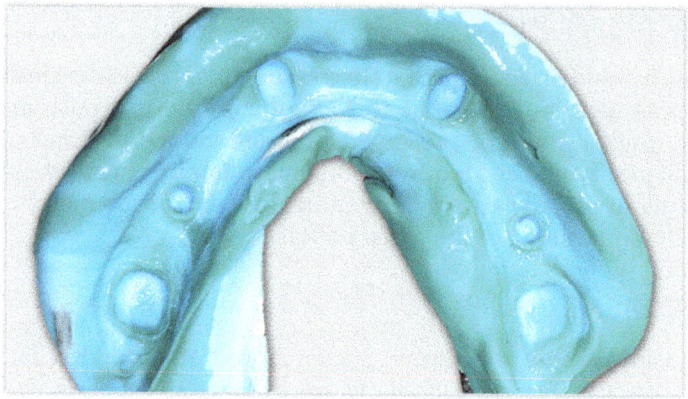

Fig. 12.3: Direct impression recording the position of the implant as well as the prepared teeth.

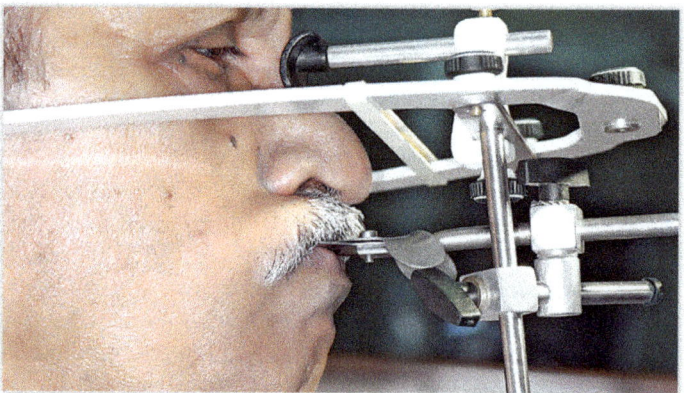

Fig. 12.4: Facebow transfer.

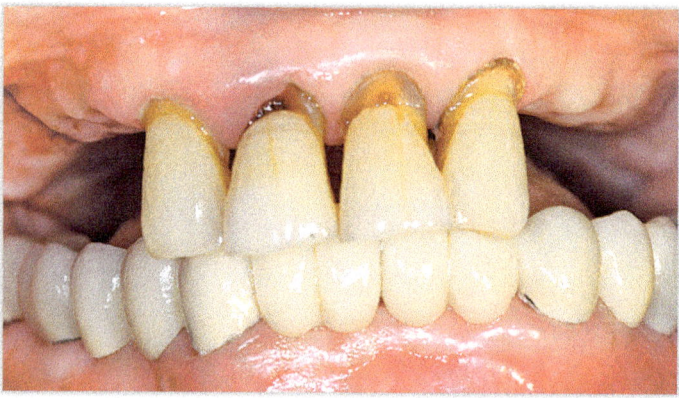

Fig. 12.5A: Ceramo-metal bridge cemented.

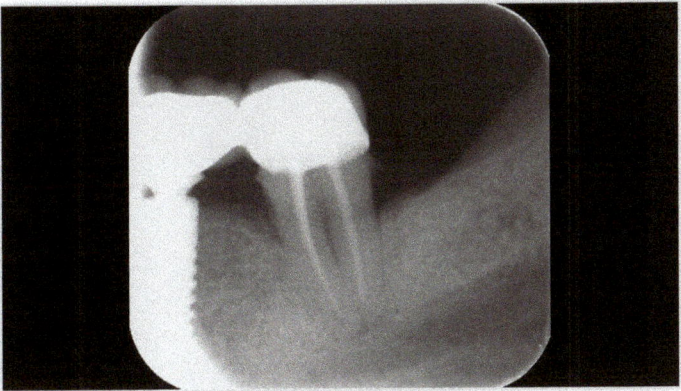

Fig. 12.5B: 10 year-follow-up

Case has a follow-up after 10 years which shows stable results except for periodontal lesion in lower left second molar which had to be treated with open flap and debridement but no peri-implantitis. Literature tells us that it is possible to connect natural teeth with implants in selected cases if you have a strong and stable implant abutment connection like that of the Ankylos implant used in this case (Dentsply Sirona) (Fig. 12.5B)

CASE 2

Challenge: High End Esthetics

Female aged 35 years reports with pain and swelling of her upper right central incisor. On examination it is found that it is an endodontically treated tooth with a crown.

TREATMENT PLAN

After explaining to the patient the various lines of treatment she could opt for, she decided to extract the tooth and go in for immediate implantation and provisional restoration.

TREATMENT

The tooth was extracted as atraumatically as possible using periotomes, thin luxators and finally a fine beaked forceps with rotational movement (Fig. 12.6). The socket was gently curetted of all granulation tissue and a purchase point made with a thin precision drill in the apical part of the palatal wall of the socket (Power Point Pilot Drill, Salvin Dental USA) (Fig. 12.7). The osteotomy was sequentially enlarged using Lindemann side cutting drill at the expense of the palatal wall (Fig. 12.8). It was further expanded by using the 3.5 mm and the 4.5 mm twist drills (Fig. 12.9). Note the original socket is bypassed and a new site for implant is created in the palatal part of the socket. The proper depth, primary

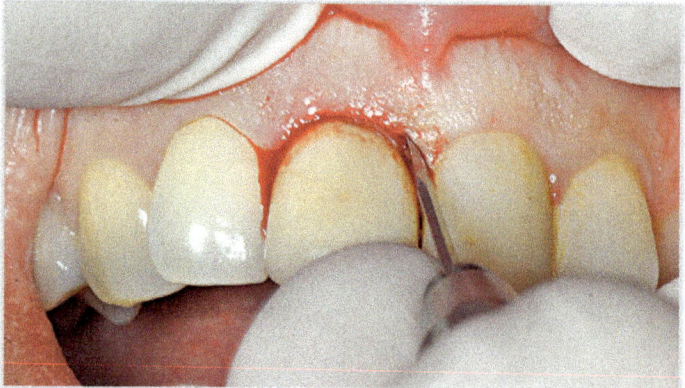

Fig. 12.6: Periotome in use for atraumatic extraction.

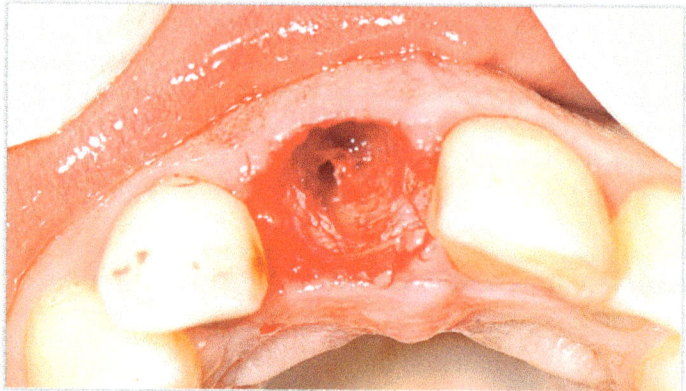

Fig. 12.7: Power Point drill marking the palatal one-third of the socket.

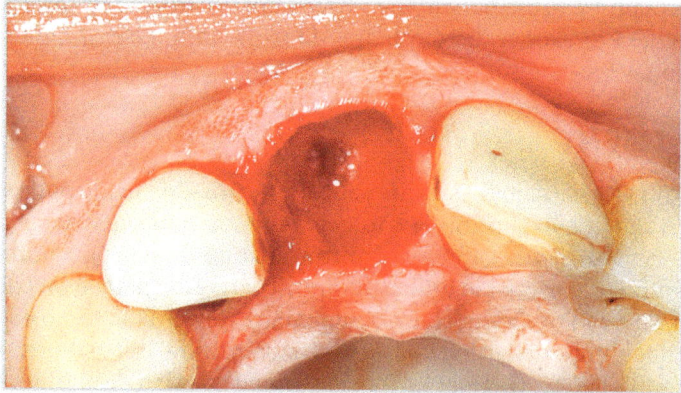

Fig. 12.8: Sequential use of Lindemann drill.

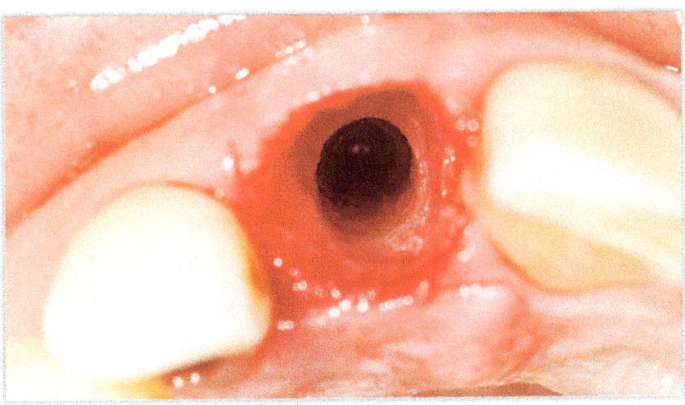

Fig. 12.9: Final osteotomy prepared in the palatal wall.

stability and correct 3D placement are checked with the conical reamer placed with the help of the Nentwig Ustomed instrument (Fig. 12.10). The site was not tapped but the Ankylos 4.5 mm implant was rotated inside the osteotomy using the motor at a speed of 15 rpm and a maximum torque of 50 Ncm taking care to use a firm hand in guiding the implant against the palatal wall of the osteotomy (Fig. 12.11). Since there remained a horizontal space of more than 2 mm from the buccal bony plate, the area was grafted and supported by a slow resorbing biomaterial Bio-Oss.[2] No membrane was placed as the mucoperiosteal flap was not raised (Fig. 12.12). A straight Balance abutment with gingival height of 3 mm was torqued in using only hand pressure (Fig. 12.13). A crown and bridge impression using alginate impression material (Jeltrate Chromatic, Dentsply Sirona) was made. A model in quick setting stone plaster was poured and a provisional in composite was sculpted on the model and cemented with a noneugenol containing temporary cement (TempBond NE, kerr Corp. USA) (Fig. 12.14). After waiting for a period of 3 months for osseointegration the titanium abutment was removed and a zirconia abutment (Cercon, Dentsply Sirona, Germany) was torqued in at 15 Ncm (Figs. 12.15 and 12.16). Since the patient was very particular for high end esthetics, the left central incisor was prepared for a porcelain veneer to match the right central incisor implant crown exactly. The veneer and the crown were prepared in lithium disilicate (Ivoclar Vivadent, Germany). Note the excellent esthetic final outcome (Fig. 12.17). Intraoral radiograph exhibits excellent marginal fit and growth of bone over the implant shoulder (Fig. 12.18).

DISCUSSION

In a highly esthetic zone it is important to preserve both hard and soft tissues. Especially preservation of the buccal cortical plate and preventing its resorption is very important. Since typically the implant is placed against the palatal wall of the socket it is essential to place a very slowly resorbing bone substitute. The above case's exceptional esthetics amply supports the above philosophy.

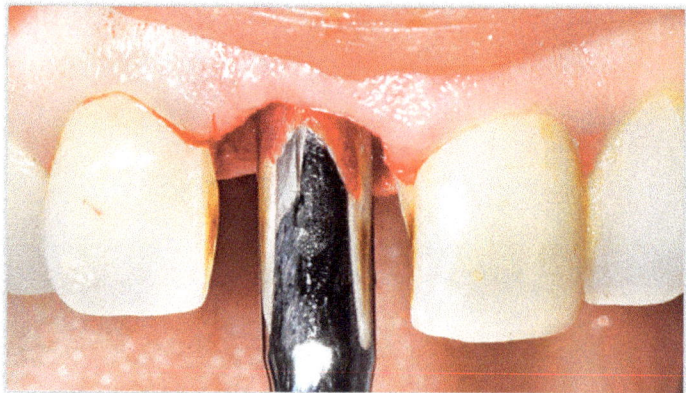

Fig. 12.10: Reamer used with Nentwig instrument.

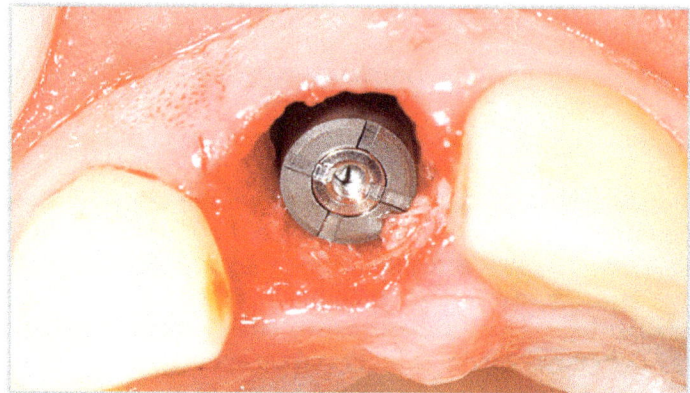

Fig. 12.11: Implant placed against palatal wall of the socket.

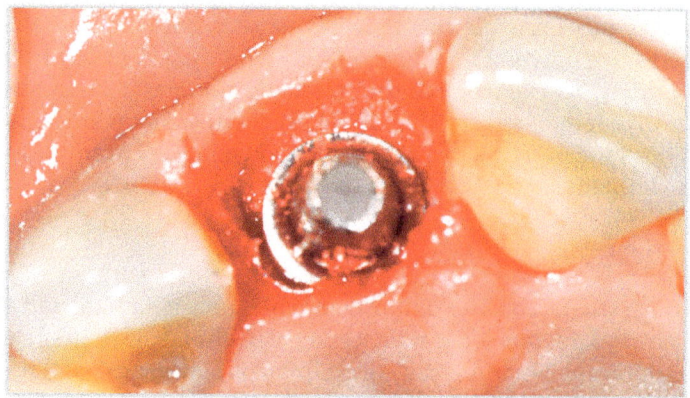

Fig. 12.12: Bio-Oss placed to support and preserve buccal wall.

Challenging Implant Cases and Their Management

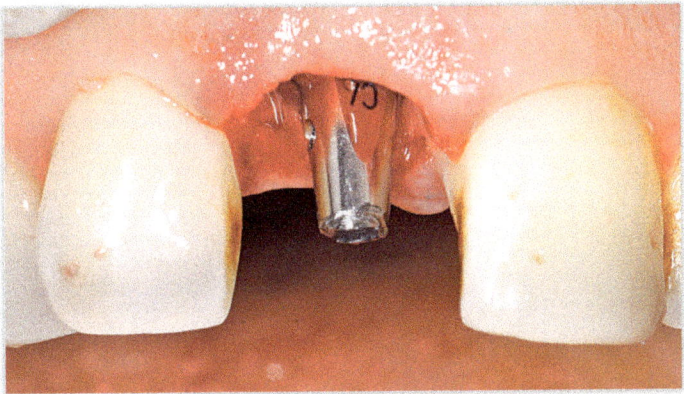

Fig. 12.13: Balance straight abutment 3.0GH.

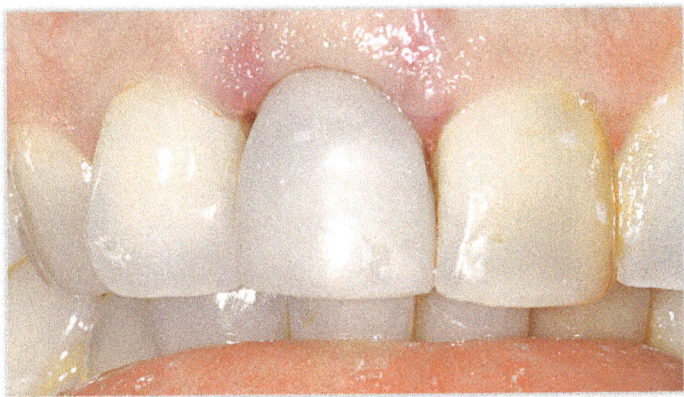

Fig. 12.14: Composite crown temporarily cemented.

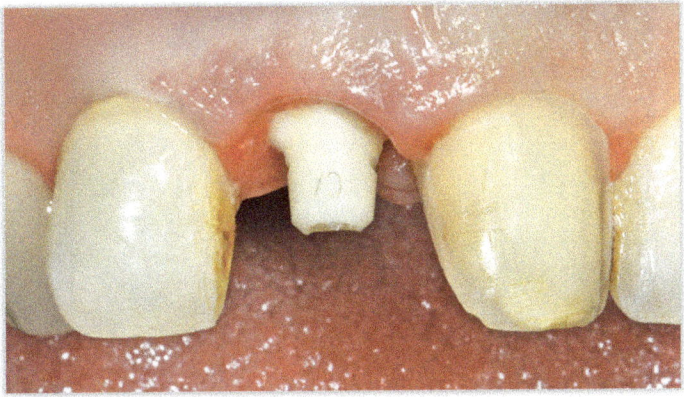

Fig. 12.15: Zirconia abutment (Cercon Denstply Sirona) torqued in at 15 Ncm. Left central incisor has been prepared for porcelain laminate veneer.

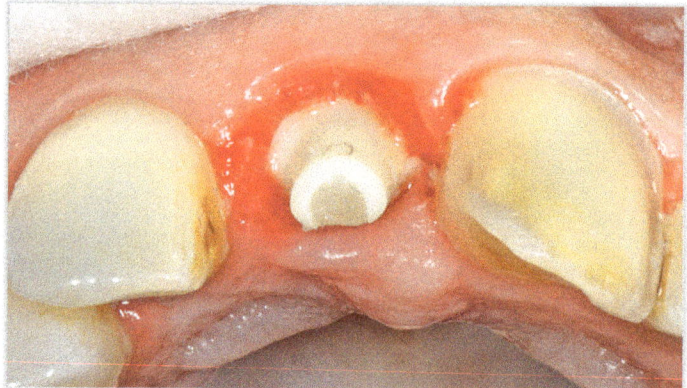

Fig. 12.16: Occlusal view of abutment and prepared veneer.

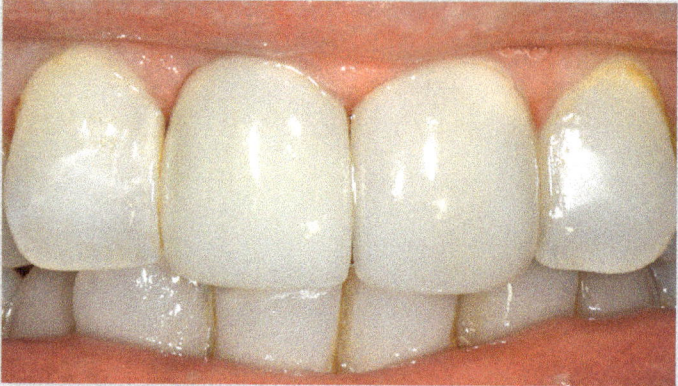

Fig. 12.17: Final all ceramic crown cemented on Cercon abutment.

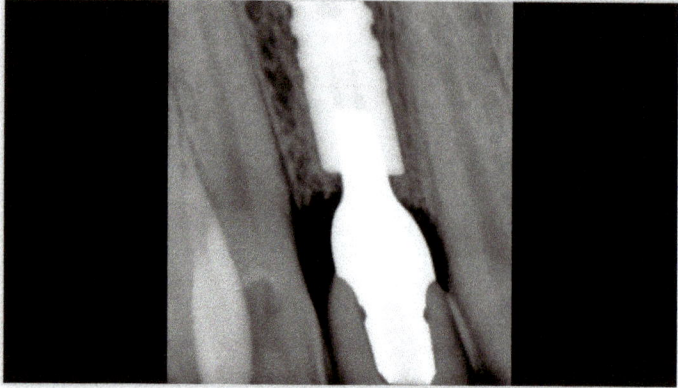

Fig. 12.18: Intraoral radiograph exhibiting excellent crestal bone preservation. Note bone has actually grown over implant the shoulder.

CASE 3

Challenge: Immediate Implantation in Absence of Buccal Plate of Bone

Although it is true that in most cases implant placement should be postponed if the buccal plate of bone is absent especially so in the critical anterior part of the maxilla; this should not be an absolute contraindication.

A male aged 60 years came to the dental office with a chief complaint of a fractured endodontically treated left central incisor (Fig. 12.19) and requested fast rehabilitation with a fixed restoration. The option was given to him for a tooth supported fixed prosthesis or an implant supported crown. He chose the latter in view of his experience with fracture of the endodontically treated tooth. Intraoral and OPG X-rays revealed no major periapical disease.

Treatment Plan

Intraoral examination revealed a very thin buccal plate of bone. It was therefore decided to do implant placement palatally and graft if buccal plate was absent. In order to preserve blood supply from the periosteum it was decided to do a flapless surgery. In view of the fact that the buccal plate would need to be grafted it was decided not to place a provisional restoration immediately after extraction but a removable acrylic partial denture was fabricated with an ovate pontic to place pressure on the marginal tissues and prevent them from collapsing.

Treatment

The root was very carefully extracted using initially microsurgical blade (Swann Morton, UK) to incise the periosteum followed by periotomes (Medesy, Italy) and finally very thin luxators (Directa, Sweden) (Fig. 12.20). Pressure by these instruments was only given mesiodistally. Buccolingual pressure was avoided with a hope of preserving the facial plate.

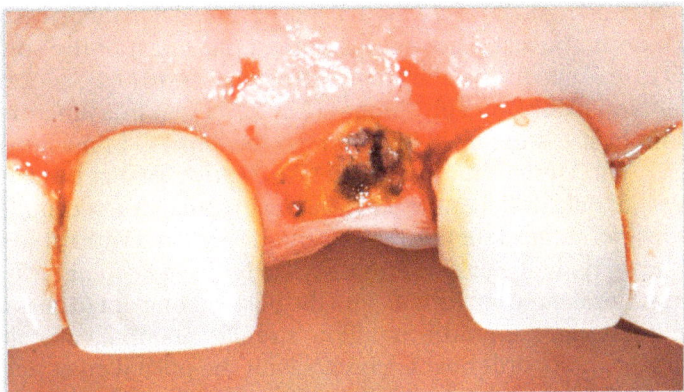

Fig. 12.19: Preoperative intraoral view.

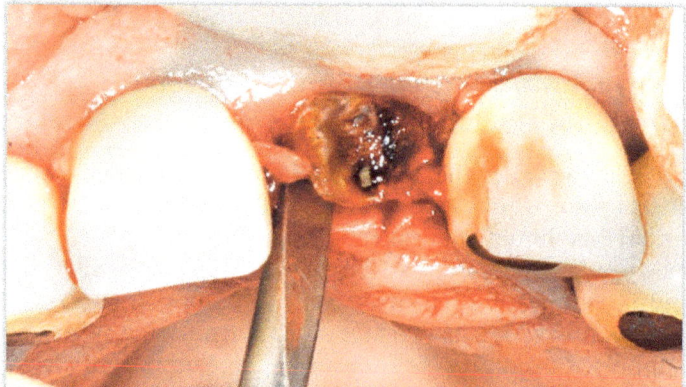

Fig. 12.20: Use of Luxator.

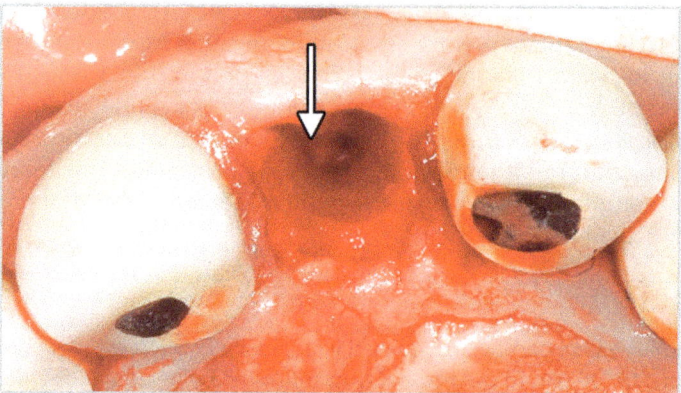

Fig. 12.21: Positioning of the initial osteotomy in the apical 1/3 of the palatal wall.

However, on removal of the tooth it was observed that there was a complete absence of the buccal plate except in the apical part of the socket. It was decided to drill into the palatal bone in the apical 1/3rd of the socket first using a Lindemann drill (Dentsply Sirona) (Fig. 12.21). At this juncture, it is very important to stress the need of a through the lens (TTL) magnifying loopes with LED light (Designs for Vision, USA) to clearly visualize the socket and be able to accurately drill into the palatal apical 1/3rd of the socket. The use of a good powerful surgical suction (Durr Dental, Germany) with a thin disposable suction tip (Friadent Roeko, Germany) also helps in keeping field bloodless. Care must be taken when drilling into the palatal bone not to go too deep, but after initial drilling, the drill should be straightened to go apically with the coronal part of the drill now in contact with the palatal crest (Fig. 12.22). It was decided to use a 4.5 mm wide and 14 mm long Ankylos implant (Dentsply Sirona). The osteotomy was sequentially enlarged always keeping the drills in

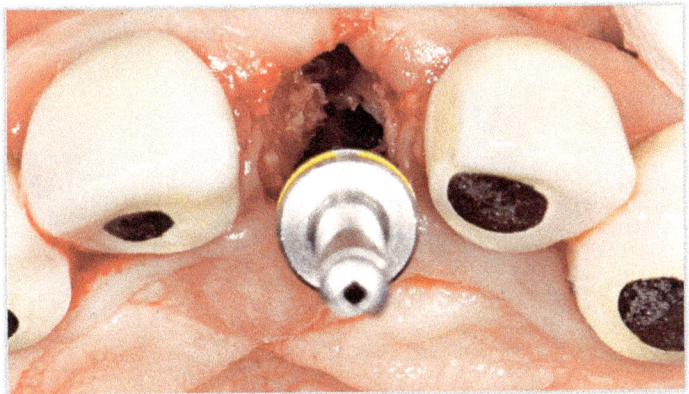

Fig. 12.22: Coronal part of the drill now in contact with the palatal crest.

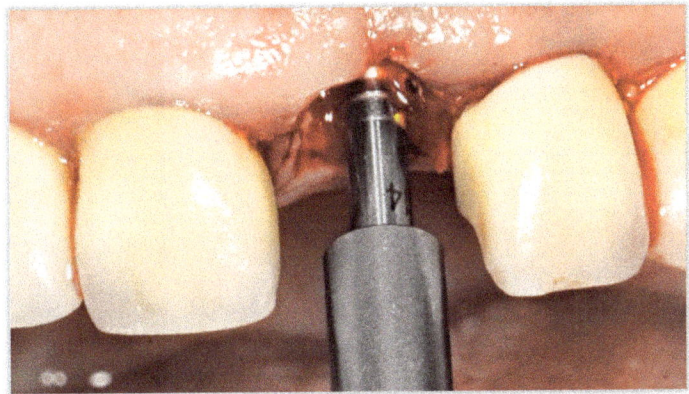

Fig. 12.23: Conical reamer demonstrating good primary stability.

contact with the palatal bone. A very useful part of the 'Ankylos' surgical kit is the conical reamer which allows you to judge how stable your implant will be on placement (Fig. 12.23). The implant was placed with the motor, again taking care to see that it was in contact with the palatal bone (Fig. 12.24). Since, it was placed palatally, the rather large defect present on the labial aspect was grafted with de-proteinized bovine bone material (DBBM) (Bio-Oss, Geistlich, Switzerland) (Fig. 12.25).[2] The edges of the wound were approximated with a figure of eight suture using 3.0 Vicryl (Johnson & Johnson, USA) (Fig. 12.26). The patient was instructed to wear the removable acrylic partial denture as minimally as possible. Note the excellent healing of the ridge and preservation of the buccal contour one month after implantation and grafting of the missing buccal plate (Fig. 12.27).

It is the opinion of the authors that the good healing without infection of the grafted material is due to the strict instruction to rinse with chlorhexidine

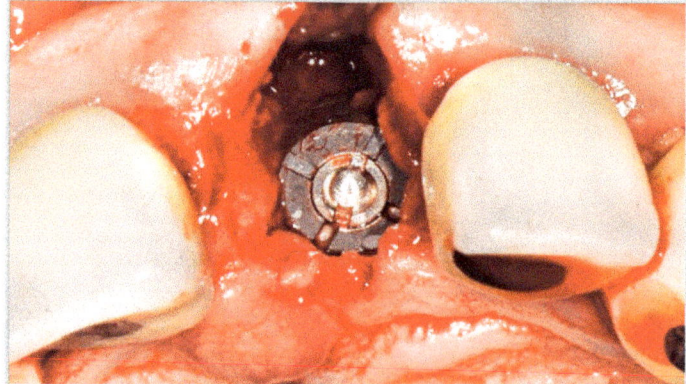

Fig. 12.24: Implant placed. Observe total absence of buccal wall.

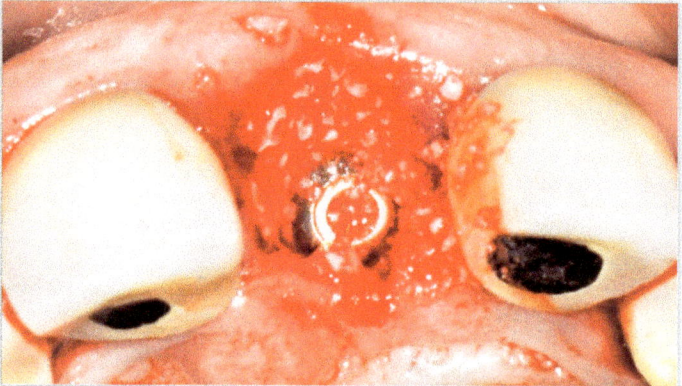

Fig. 12.25: Grafting of the buccal wall with DBBM (Bio-Oss).

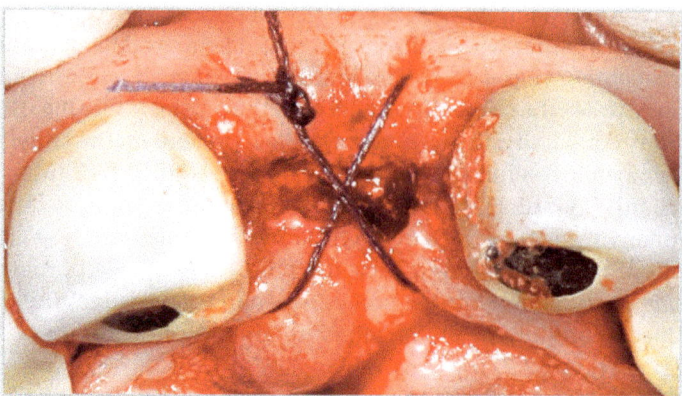

Fig. 12.26: Closing of the wound with a figure of eight suture.

Challenging Implant Cases and Their Management

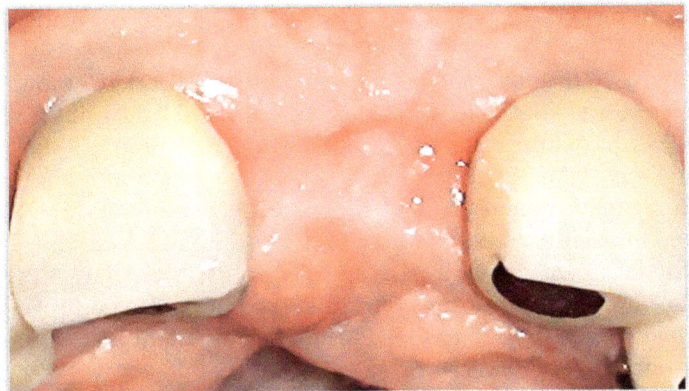

Fig. 12.27: Excellent wound healing after 1 month of surgery showing preservation of buccal contour.

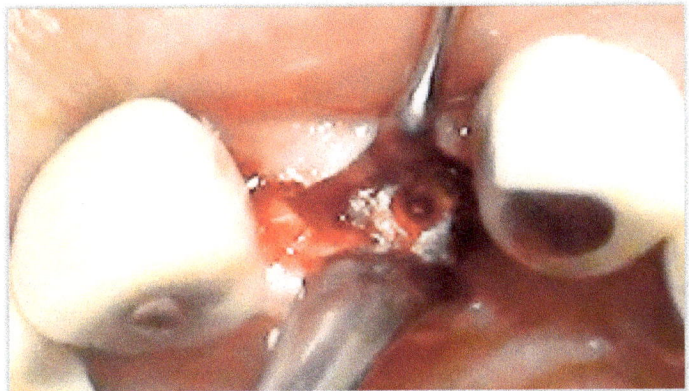

Fig. 12.28: Keyhole stage II surgery showing uncovery of implant.

gluconate 0.12% in alcohol base (Periogard, Colgate Palmolive India) three times a day keeping the solution for 30 seconds in the mouth starting on the day of surgery and continued for 15 days. After a period of 3 months, the second stage surgery is commenced by means of key hole surgery which is possible with the 'Ankylos' implant system because of conical implant abutment connection (Fig. 12.28). The advantages of minimal reflection of the flap are that DBBM (Bio-Oss) is not disturbed and the tissues are minimally damaged. At this stage the final abutment was torqued in at only 15 Ncm which is the recommended torque for Ankylos abutments. The abutment was reshaped outside the mouth using tungsten carbide burs (SS White USA). They were finally finished and polished using Enhance and Pogo discs (Dentsply Sirona). A crown and bridge impression in alginate (Jeltrate Chromatic, Dentsply Sirona) was taken and a cast in stone plaster (Ultrastone, Kalabhai Dental) was poured.

A temporary crown was custom made in the clinic by using the Duo shades of Ceram-X Duo (Dentsply Sirona) (Fig. 12.29). The crowns were slightly overcontoured to support the soft tissue. After a period of 3 months the final PFM crown was fabricated by taking a crown and bridge impression using Aquasil Ultra L.V. and Aquasil soft putty (Dentsply Sirona) in a single stage one step procedure. The final PFM was cemented on the abutment using a resin modified glass ionomer cement (Rely.X luting cement, 3M ESPE). Note the good red and white esthetics in the severely compromised case. The contact points of the crown were shifted as apically as possible to reduce their distance from the interproximal crestal bone; this was done with a hope of regeneration of the lost papilla (Fig. 12.30).[3] IOPA showing excellent crestal bone levels as well as perfect fit of PFM crown. (Fig. 12.31)

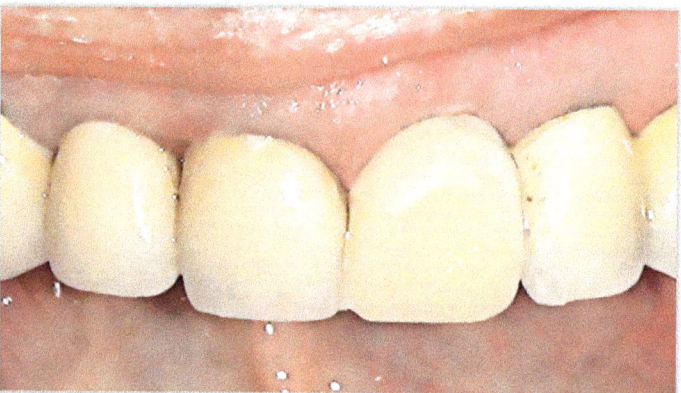

Fig. 12.29: After 3 months permanent balance abutment is torqued in and a provisional is temporarily cemented to sculpt the tissues.

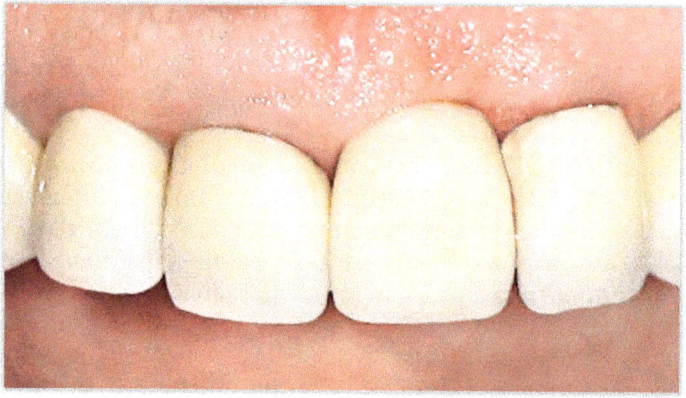

Fig. 12.30: After 1 month for stabilization of soft tissues the permanent PFM crown is cemented.

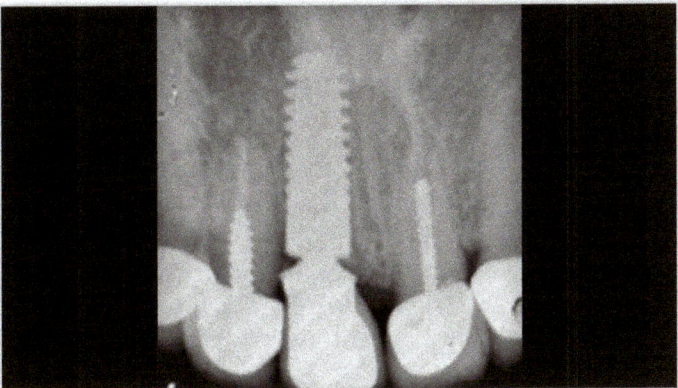

Fig. 12.31: IOPA showing excellent crestal bone levels as well as perfect fit of PFM crown.

DISCUSSION

In retrospect and summarizing the case, the reasons we got the fairly high esthetic result in a severely compromised case where there was complete loss of buccal cortical bone was possible due to following steps employed:
- Atraumatic extraction of tooth causing least damage to hard and soft tissue.
- Flapless implant placement to preserve blood supply for tissue regeneration.
- Drilling at the expense of the palatal cortical bone of the socket and completely bypassing the original socket. Also going about 3 mm apical to root socket.
- Obtaining adequate primary stability with the above protocol.
- Grafting and supporting the buccal soft tissue devoid of buccal plate of bone by using a well-documented bone substitute like 'Bio-Oss'(Geistlich) without a membrane. The mucoperiosteum which was not reflected acted like a membrane and profused the biomaterial with blood supply. The other advantage of using Bio-Oss is its rather limited and slow resorption which helped in supporting the buccal contour of the ridge. Using autogenous bone in this situation with its fast resorption would not have been a better alternative.
- Allowing implant to remain submerged without loading with a provisional and protecting the bone substitute from getting infected by using antibiotics for 5 days and chlorhexidine rinses (Periogard, Colgate) for 15 days.
- Keyhole surgery at the second stage to prevent disturbance of maturing bone substitute and minimizing gingival recession.
- Torquing in the abutment only once and no frequent attachment—reattachment of components on the implant. This helped in preventing disruption of the connective tissue attachment on the implant.

Using the well documented "Ankylos" implant system with the conical tapered abutment which allows minimal trauma during second stage surgery. It also preserves hard and soft tissues because of:
- Platform shifting.
- No micromovement and no microbial growth between implant and abutment due to cold welding of the attachment.
- Support of soft tissues due to the conical taper of the abutment.

Reshaping support and maturation of the soft tissues by fabrication of a custom made provisional with a biocompatible and highly polishable composite (Ceram-X Duo, Dentsply Sirona).

Excellent support and back up from the dental lab (Adaro Dental Labs, Mumbai)

CASE 4

Challenge: Implant Placement Avoiding the Anterior Loop of Mandibular Nerve

Male aged 54 years reports to the dental clinic with paresthesia in lower right side of the mandible. He gives a history of implant placement in the region about 2 years back. The implant had to be removed the next day after surgery with the help of an oral surgeon, since, the dentist knew he had injured the inferior alveolar nerve whilst placement of the implant. Since, that time he has numbness and altered sensation in that area. He requests rehabilitation of his right second premolar and first molar with a fixed prosthesis.

TREATMENT PLAN

After doing a thorough intraoral examination, OPG and CT scan it is observed that the available height of bone is only 9 mm from the crest of the ridge to the inferior alveolar nerve (Fig. 12.32). It was therefore decided to drill only

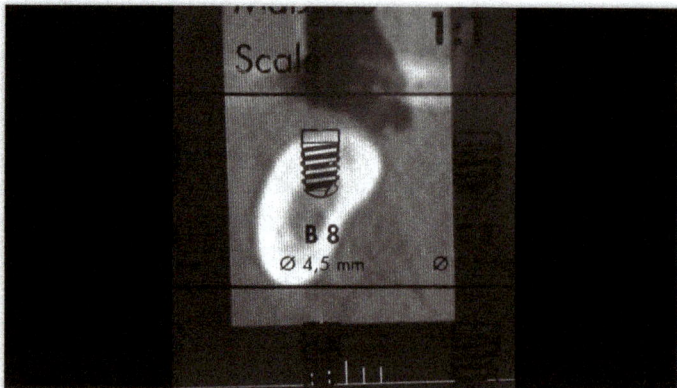

Fig. 12.32: Bone height measured.

up to 7 mm and take an intraoral digital X-ray and if enough height from the inferior alveolar canal is present then we would drill to 8 mm and place two Ankylos A8 implants.

TREATMENT

A midcrestal incision was made with sulcular incisions in the canine, first premolar and second molar region. The mucoperiosteal flap was reflected and the mental nerve was identified (Fig. 12.33). Care was taken to drill posterior to the mental foramen thus avoiding injury to it. The mental foramen in this case was situated more coronally than the inferior alveolar canal (Fig. 12.34). This was probably the reason for injury of the mental nerve by the previous dentist. After drilling to a depth of 7 mm with the pilot drill a digital intraoral X-ray taken showed that we had about 3-4 mm more height from the inferior alveolar canal (Fig. 12.35). It was therefore decided to drill to the full depth of 8 mm in the two osteotomies and place two Ankylos A8 implants (Figs. 12.36A and 12.36B). The patient reported no complications the next day. After waiting for a period of 3 months, bone training (Progressive bone loading) was started after placing two abutments and making two splinted composite crowns (Fig. 12.37). After bone training for six weeks final zirconia all ceramic crowns were cemented (Figs. 12.38A and12.38B)

DISCUSSION

The case amply exemplifies the need to identify carefully the mental foramen. However, it must be clarified that one must be extremely gentle to avoid traumatizing the mental nerve while exposing it. The anterior loop of the mental foramen has been reported frequently in the literature and in this case due to the loop the mental foramen was shifted considerably coronally with the result unless it was identified the possibility of injuring it during osteotomy preparation is large.

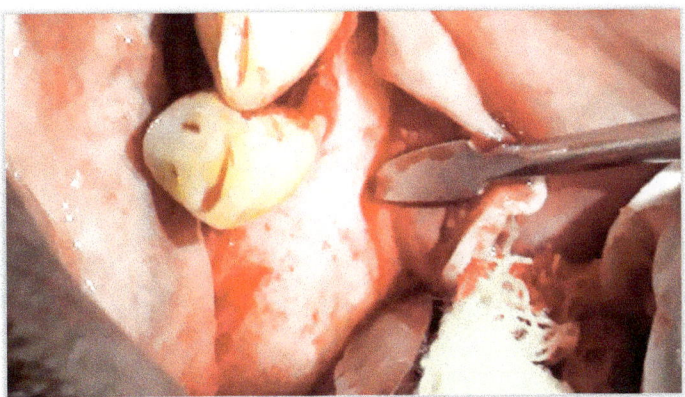

Fig. 12.33: Identification of mental foramen.

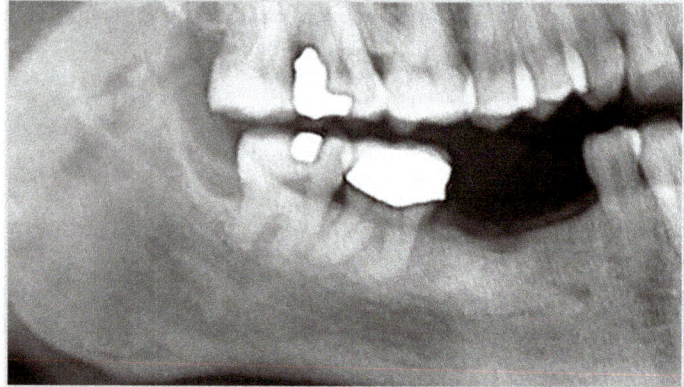

Fig. 12.34: Mental foramen coronal to the inferior alveolar canal.

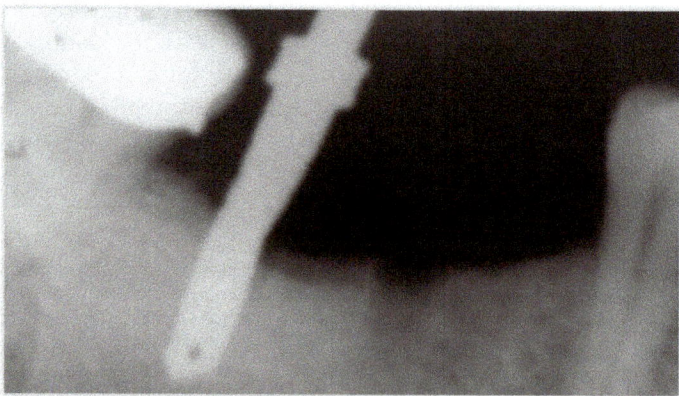

Fig. 12.35: Intraoral X-ray after initial drilling.

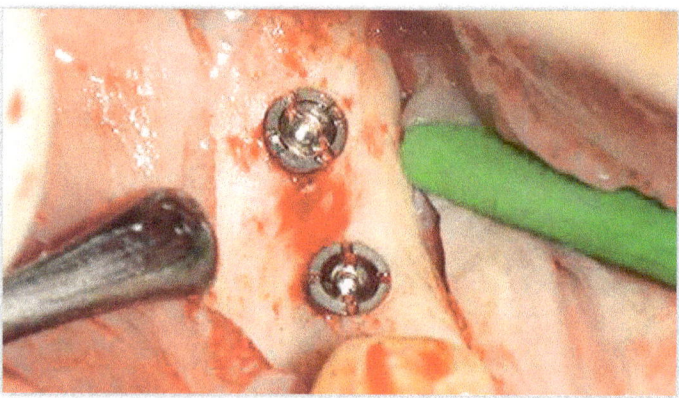

Fig. 12.36A: Two A8 implants placed.

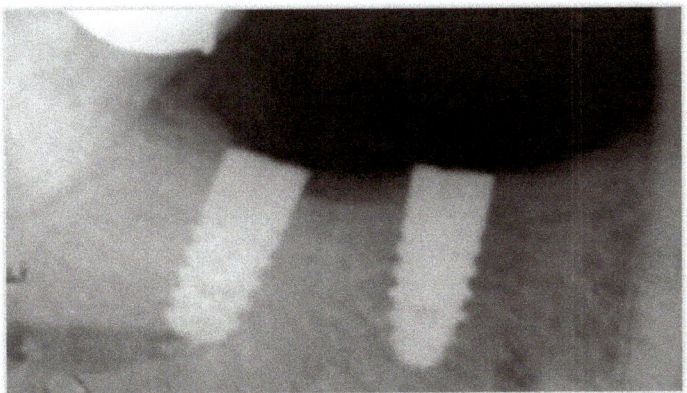

Fig. 12.36B: Radiograph of the two implant after placement.

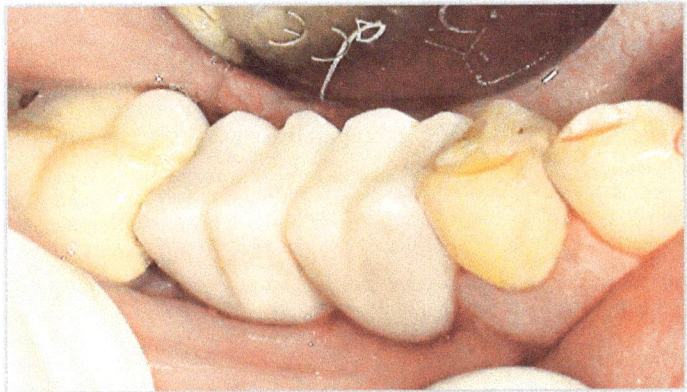

Fig. 12.37: Temporary crowns placed 3 months after implant placement for bone training

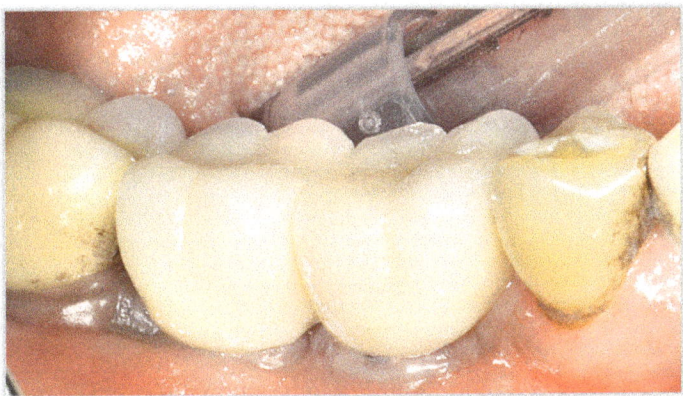

Fig. 12.38A: Note good marginal fit and esthetics.

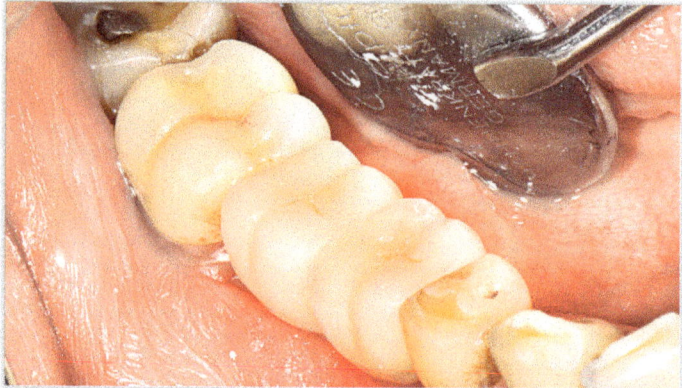

Fig. 12.38B: Occlusal view of the zirconia all ceramic crowns.

REFERENCES

1. Gross M, Abramovich I, Weiss EI. Microleakage at the abutment-implant interface of osseointegrated implants: a comparative study. Int J Oral Maxillofac Implants. 1999;14(1):94-100.
2. Araújo MG, Linder E, Lindhe J. Bio-Oss collagen in the buccal gap at immediate implants: a 6-month study in the dog. Clin Oral Implants Res. 2011;22(1):1-8
3. Tarnow DP, Magner AW, Fletcher P. The effect of the distance from the contact point to the crest of bone on the presence or absence of the interproximal dental papilla. J Periodontol. 1992;63(12):995-6.

Chapter 13

Complications After Implant Placement

Today more and more dentists are choosing implant therapy over conventional method of tooth replacement, correspondingly a rise in the number of complications related to biology, technical and aesthetic have been reported. Consequently, the importance of treating complications such as peri-implant infections is increasing. Follow-up studies have shown that the prevalence of peri-implantitis ranges from 12 to 40% for some implant systems. Fortunately, it is rare with the Ankylos Implant system. Methods of diagnosis, etiology and risk factors have been identified in a number of experimental and clinical studies done recently by many workers. In addition, a number of non-surgical, surgical, and regenerative therapies have been suggested in the management of peri-implantitis. Unfortunately, a few cases of peri-implantitis even after aggressive treatment fail to resolve often leading to explantation. Newer therapeutic modalities have, however, prevented progression of infection in most cases and given new hope that patients with peri-implantitis will be able to retain their implant borne prosthesis for long term. Although many of these complications are patient-related meaning lack of patients healing response, non-compliance of oral hygiene and maintenance recalls; a few are due to iatrogenic factors (complications due to errors by the dentist). The clinician is responsible for carrying out best possible treatment using appropriate biomaterials with the least risk and morbidity to the patient.

The clinical cases presented in this chapter cover the range of problems and complications that can occur. The first case is a case of peri-implantitis and tissue destruction after immediate implantation due to elastomeric impression material inadvertently left behind. The second case is due to overheating of bone due to placement of implant at high speed. The third case is related to an aesthetic problem due to labial placement of an implant in the anterior maxilla.

CASE 1

Female aged 45 years was referred to the dental practice by a colleague for pain and swelling after immediate implantation and provisionalization done about one and a half months back. On clinical and radiographic examination, a tentative diagnosis of peri-implantitis was made probably due to retained cement after placement of provisional (Figs. 13.1 and 13.2). It was decided to do an open surgical debridement to localize and remove excess cement. On reflection of the buccal and palatal flaps, it was found that instead of expected cement, there was a significant amount of elastomeric impression material retained on the buccal and palatal surface round about the implant abutment connection (Figs. 13.3 and 13.4). It was also noticed that a significant amount of bone destruction had also taken place. It was therefore decided to remove the implant by turning it anticlockwise from the remaining apical bone (Figs. 13.5 and 13.6). The area was thoroughly curetted of all infected and inflamed tissue and the wound closed. The patient was put on systemic antibiotics for 5 days. After a period of 10 days, the area was again re-entered and any remaining granulation tissue was curetted and the area grafted with autogenous bone from the nasal spine mixed with deproteinized bovine

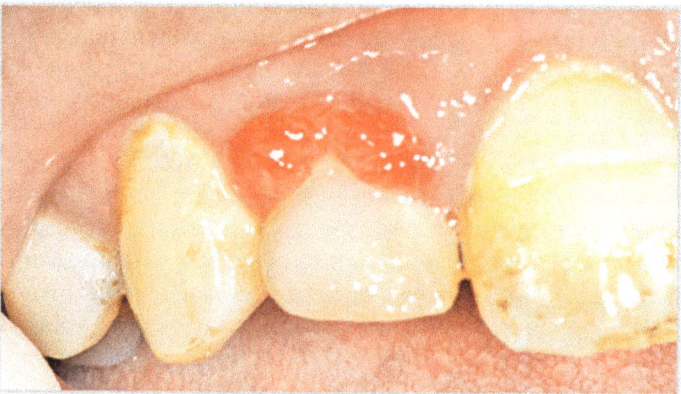

Fig. 13.1: Peri-implantitis in region of 13.

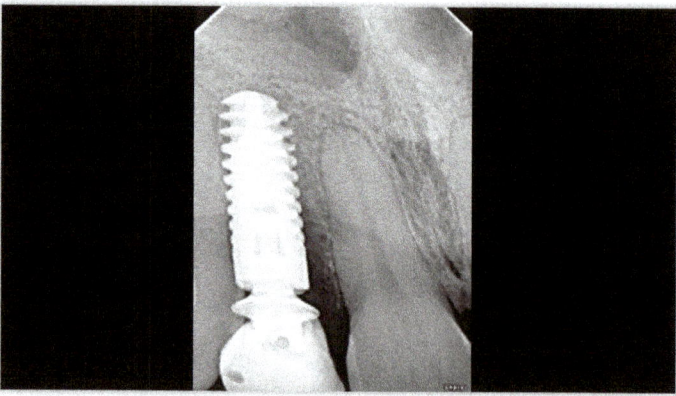

Fig. 13.2: Radiographic view of 13.

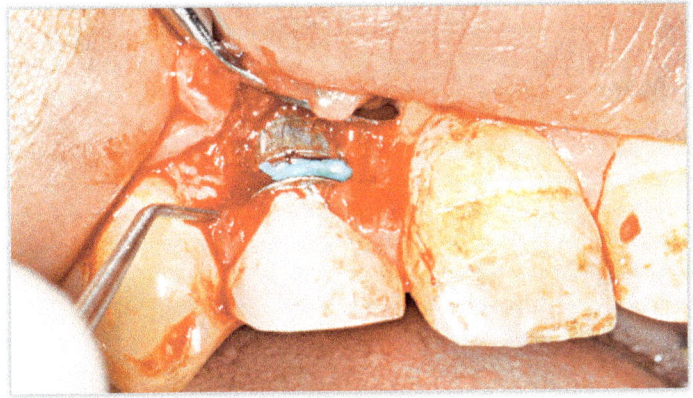

Fig. 13.3: Clinical view of retained elastomeric impression material.

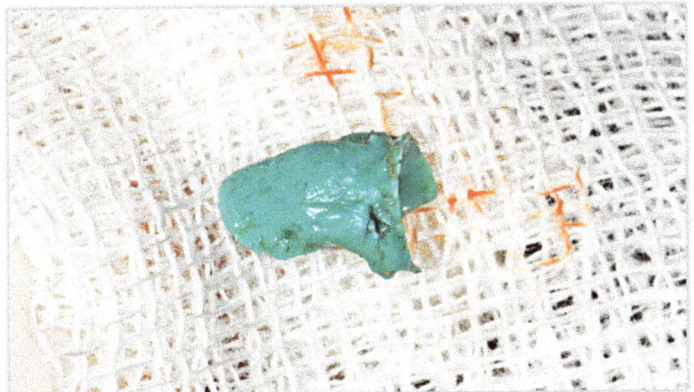

Fig. 13.4: Impression material after removal (Note considerable excess).

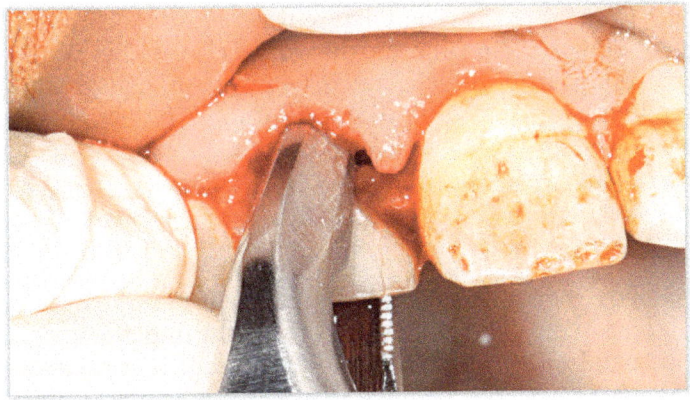

Fig. 13.5: Removal of implant with forceps.

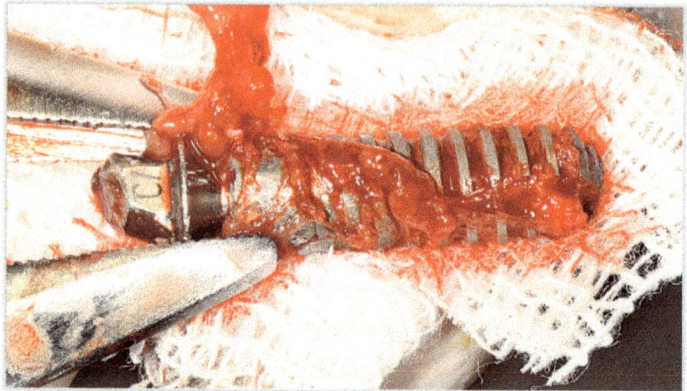

Fig. 13.6: Note destruction of bone due to peri-implantitis.

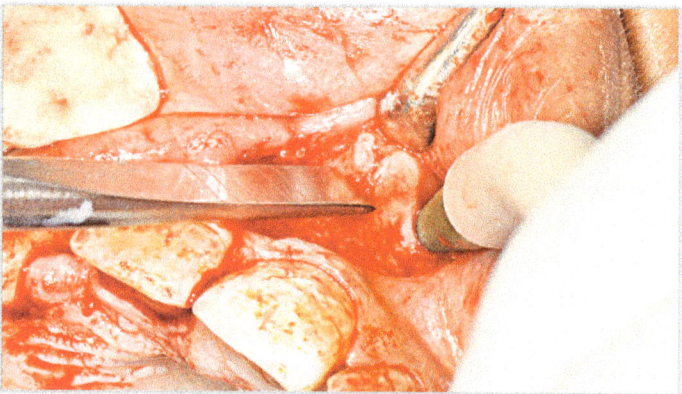

Fig. 13.7: Harvesting of bone from nasal opine with chisel.

bone Bio-Oss (Fig. 13.7). The mixture was covered with non-crosslinked collagen membrane Bio-Gide and the wound closed (Fig. 13.8). The patient was next temporarily rehabilitated with a composite resin fabricated Maryland type of fixed restoration (Fig. 13.9). The patient tolerated the procedure well and it is planned to place an implant in the grafted site after a period of 4 months.

CASE 2

Male aged 54 years was treated for placement of implant in upper right premolar region. After the initial osteotomy, the implant was placed with a motor but by mistake instead of placing it at a speed of 15 rpm, it was placed at a speed of 2000 rpm without coolant. This caused the bone to overheat and the implant failed to osseointegrate and had to be removed (Figs. 13.10 and 13.11).

Complications After Implant Placement

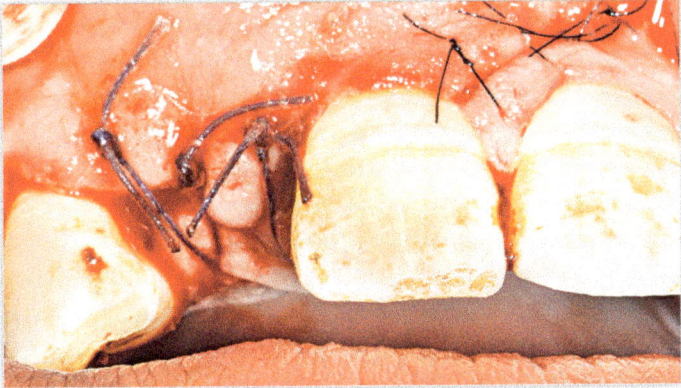

Fig. 13.8: Crestal incision closed with 4-0 vicryl and vertical incision with 5-0 nylon.

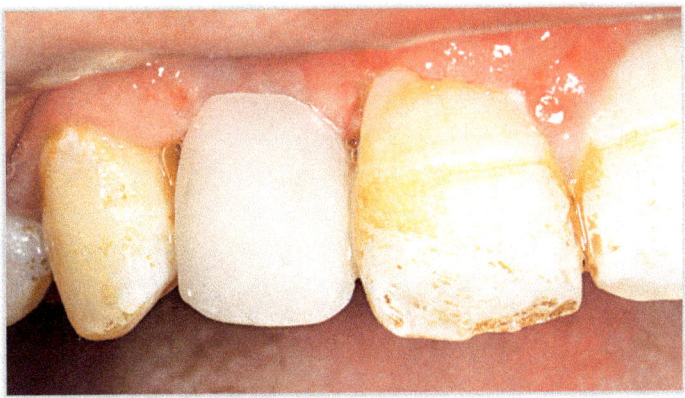

Fig. 13.9: Composite resin fabricated 12 bonded to palatal surface of adjacent teeth.

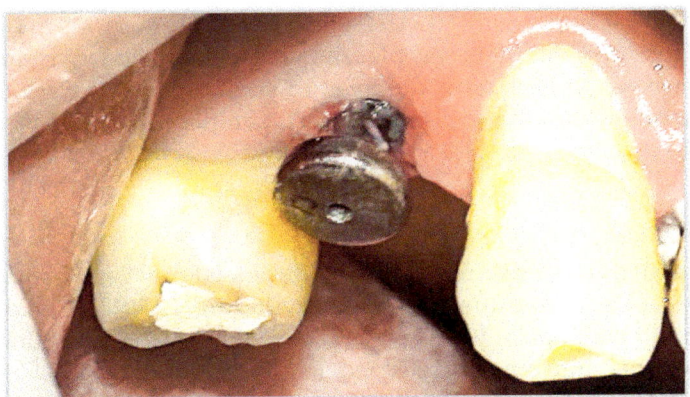

Fig. 13.10: Intraoral view of failed implant.

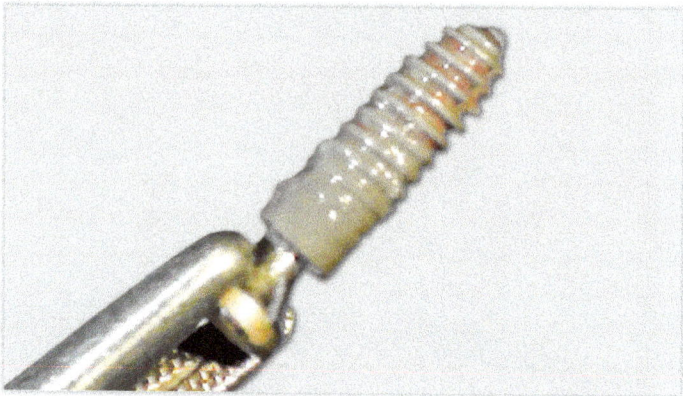

Fig. 13.11: Note brownish color of bone around the implant due to overheating.

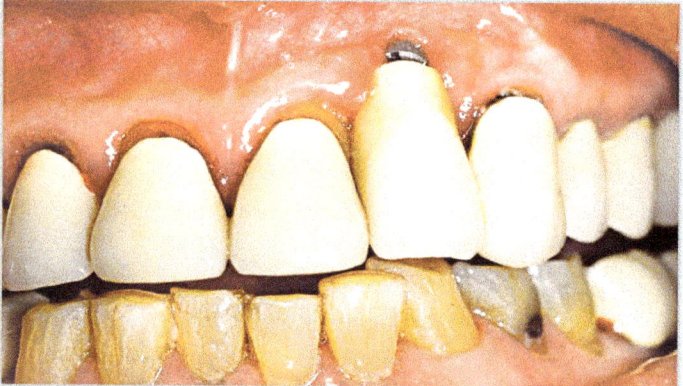

Fig. 13.12: Soft tissue recession and exposure of implant in 22.

The area was thoroughly curetted and closed. After waiting for a period of 3 months a fresh implant was placed in the same region with good results. The case report highlights the need to countercheck the speed and the setting on the motor and also to rotate the implant outside before placing it in the osteotomy site.

CASE 3

Male aged 75 years is referred by a dentist for possible soft tissue grafting because of recession and exposure of implant labially (Fig. 13.12). On examination, it was found the implant was placed too labially with the result that although the area was grafted by the referring dentist at the time of implantation, the tissue did not remain stable but was lost. Since the implant was integrated and not mobile, and since there was no inflammation or infection the patient was advised not to do anything, since there was very little chance of any soft tissue grafting being a success because there would not be any support because of lack of buccal bone. Fortunately, the patient has a long upper lip which hides the unaesthetic appearance. He was advised to keep the area clean with a soft toothbrush and report periodically for prophylaxis and check-up. The case report highlights the importance of countersinking the implant, especially in the upper anterior region in the palatal cortical bone so that guided bone regeneration can be a success.[1]

REFERENCES

1. Buser D, Martin W, Belser UC. Optimizing esthetics for implant restorations in the anterior maxilla: anatomic and surgical considerations. Int J Oral Maxillofac Implants. 2004;19.

Chapter 14

Principles of Suturing

The primary objective of dental suturing is to position and secure surgical flaps to promote healing. The sharper the incision and the less trauma inflicted on the wound, the greater the chances for primary healing. If tears or excessive damage occurs to the flaps the wound will heal by secondary intention. Sutures also aid in hemostasis. However before suturing all bleeding must be controlled, otherwise a hematoma may form underneath the flap leading to infection. Sutures help in covering the bone with the periosteal flap which is a very important function, otherwise the bone can get necrosed leading to prolonged healing.

The suture needle usually used in the oral cavity is a 3/8th circle reverse cutting edge and the suture material is either monofilament nylon (non-resorbable) or Polyglactin (PG) (resorbable). The Polyglactin suture (Vicryl, Johnson and Johnson) is the most preferred suture in a size of 4-0. However, it takes about 3–4 weeks to resorb. The advantage of PG sutures is that they are less stiff and remain tied without loosening. They are also more comfortable for the patient. They also do not wick, thus bacteria are not drawn inside the wound. The authors prefer to use 4-0 Polyglactin (Vicryl, Johnson and Johnson) for closure of most incisions in implant surgery, except the vertical releasing incision where they prefer to use 5-0 monofilament nylon (Ethicon, Johnson and Johnson) (Fig. 14.1).

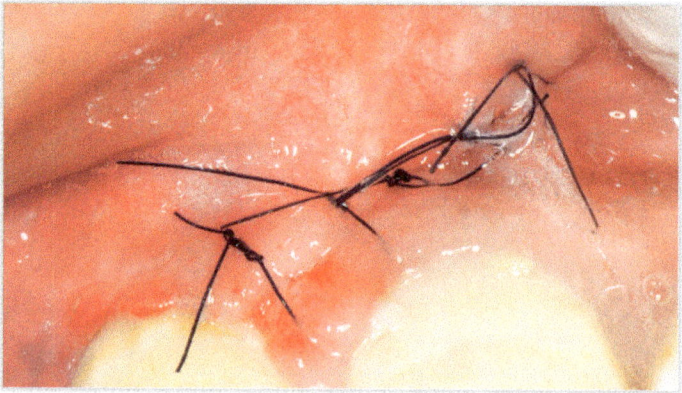

Fig. 14.1: Vertical release incision sutured with 5-0 monofilament nylon.

Principles of Suturing

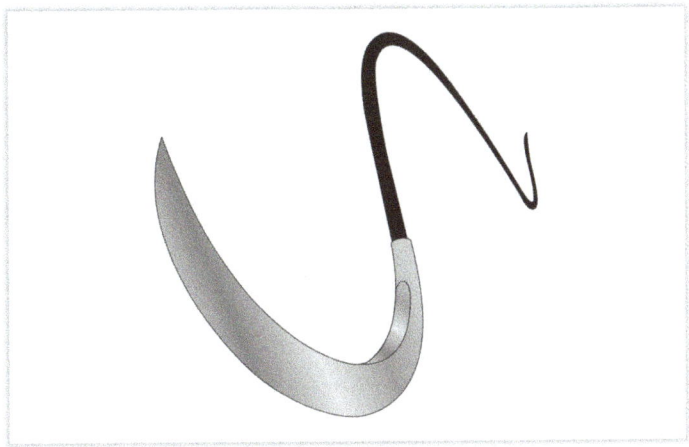

Fig. 14.2: Suture swaged to needle.

Today needles are permanently attached (swaged) to the sutures, thus eliminating the need for threading (Fig. 14.2). Silk sutures consist of silk filaments which are braided or twisted together. Although they are elastic and have knot security, they are nonresorbable and have a wick effect which causes the suture material to draw in bacteria and fluids into the wound cavity which may result in infection. They have largely been replaced by polyglycolic acid (PGA) or monofilament nylon sutures, especially in implant surgery.

SUTURING INSTRUMENTS

Various instruments are utilized in conjunction with suturing.

Tissue Forceps

These instruments must have delicate tips with teeth which serve to hold the tissues whilst sutures are passed through them. Tissue forceps must not crush or pierce tissues (Fig. 14.3).

Needle Holders

The needle holder is an instrument with a locking handle and a short beak. It should be manufactured of high quality steel with tungsten carbide inserts (Fig. 14.4). The needle holder is different from a hemostat which has a long beak and is usually used for clamping blood vessels and to grab loose objects (Fig. 14.5). Hemostats should not be used as needle holders. The needle holder grasps the needle about 1–2 minutes from the swaged end. The needle should not be grasped near its tip and cutting edges nor at the swaged end.

Scissors

A variety of scissors are available for suture cutting. The preferred suture scissor has a long handle and a short cutting edge because their sole purpose is to cut sutures (Fig. 14.6).

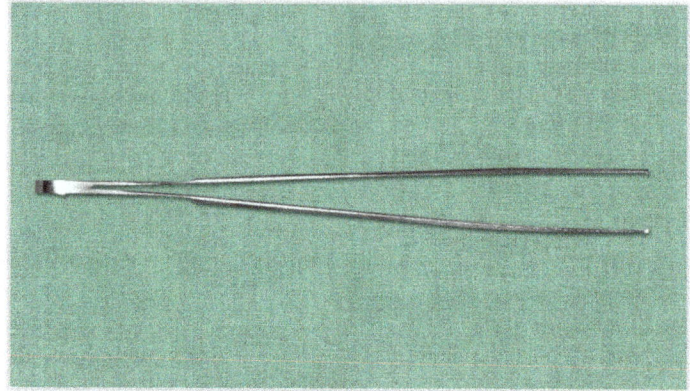

Fig. 14.3: Delicate tissue-holding forcep.

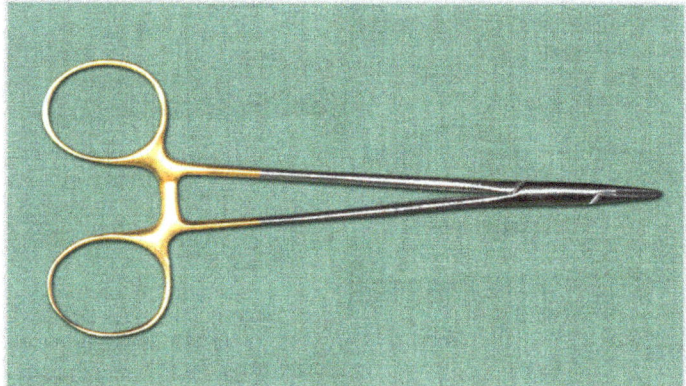

Fig. 14.4: Fine needle holder.

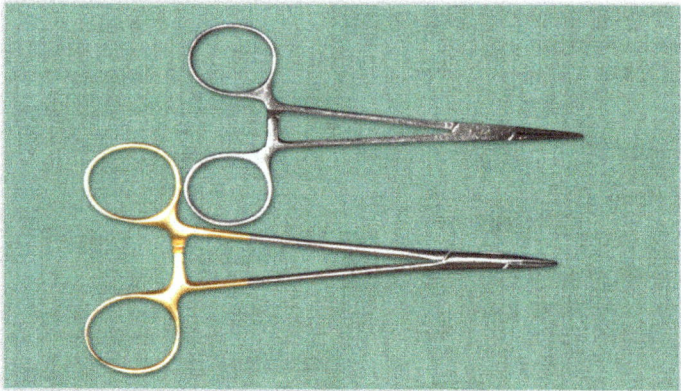

Fig. 14.5: Hemostat (Top), Needle holder (Below).

Principles of Suturing 189

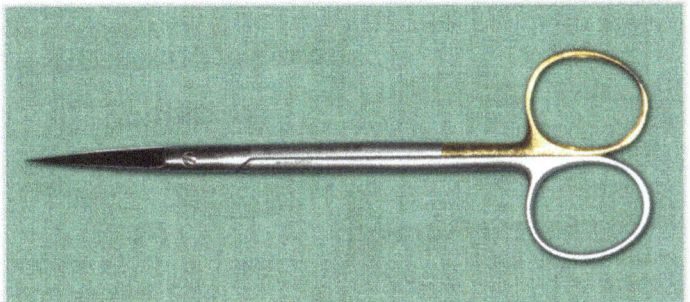

Fig. 14.6: Suture scissor.

SUTURING TECHNIQUES

Interrupted Suture Technique

The simple interrupted suture is the one most frequently used in implant surgery. The suture goes through the buccal flap, comes out through the lingual flap and is brought back and tied on the buccal side (Figs. 14.7A to D).

Modification of Interrupted Suture Technique for Interdental Areas

In this technique after entering the buccal flap the needle is passed below the contact point, but does not pass through the inner side of the lingual flap, instead it passes through the outer side of the lingual flap and then passes again below the contact point and is tied on the buccal side. The advantage is that it is easier to see the exact point of entry on the lingual side and you are not guessing (Figs. 14.8A to D).

Simple Interrupted Suture Technique (Figs. 14.7A to D)

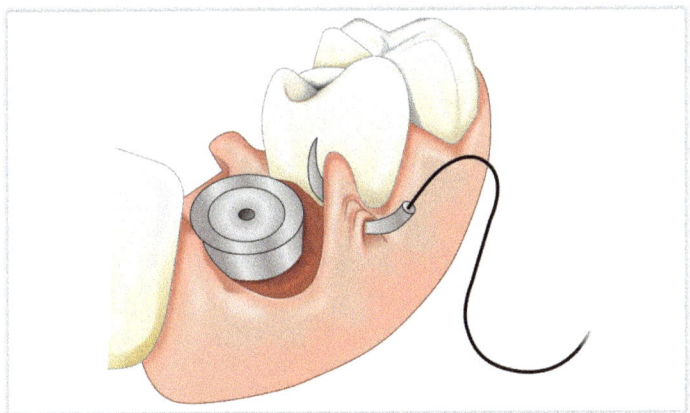

Fig. 14.7A: First needle entry from outer part of buccal flap.

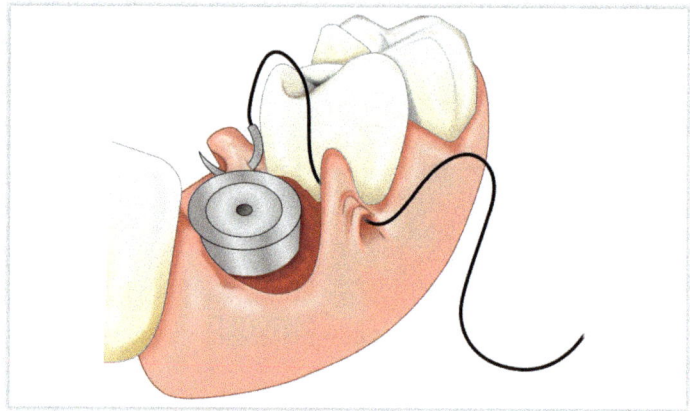

Fig. 14.7B: Needle pass underneath contact point and through inner part of lingual flap.

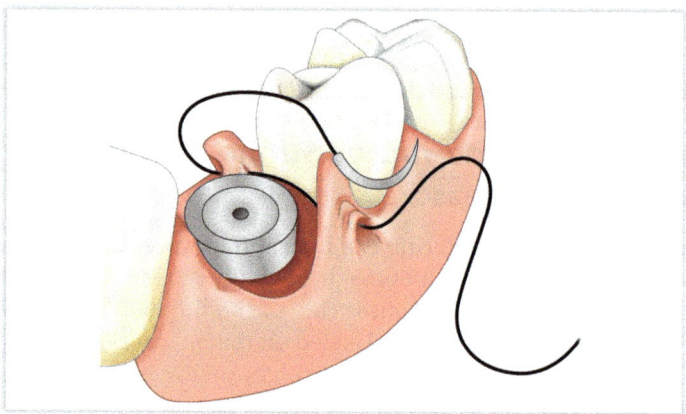

Fig. 14.7C: Needle repassed under contact point.

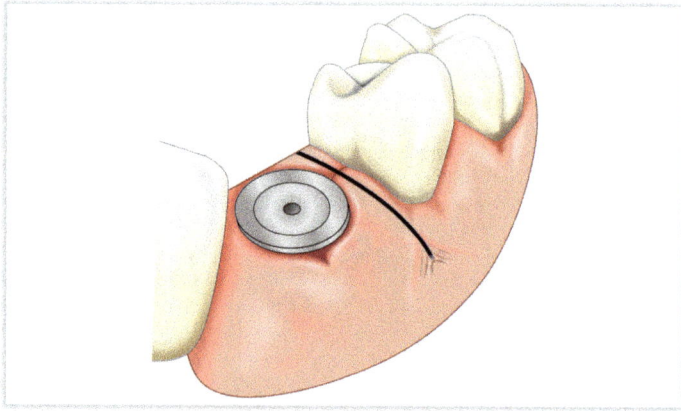

Fig. 14.7D: Knot tied on buccal side.

Modified Interrupted Suture Technique (Figs. 14.8A to D)

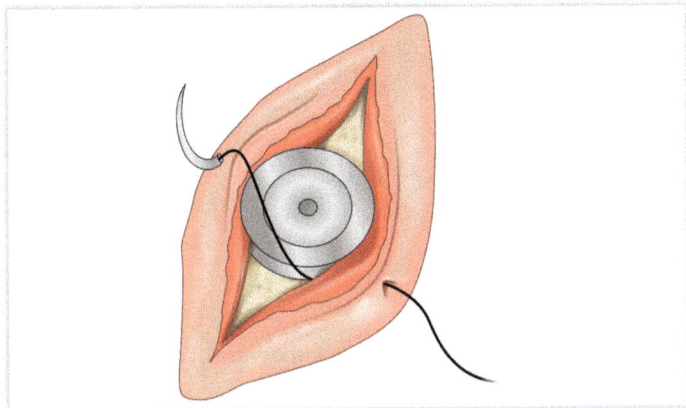

Fig. 14.8A: Entry of needle through outer side of buccal flap.

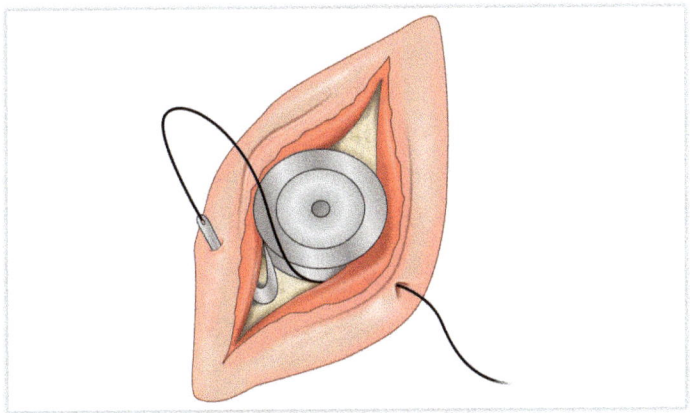

Fig. 14.8B: Needle passed underneath contact point and entered through outer side of lingual flap.

Horizontal Mattress Suture

A suturing technique which is useful for relieving tension on the incision line is the horizontal mattress suture (Figs. 14.9A to D).

Vertical Mattress Suture

The vertical mattress suture technique is used to resist tension in the flaps produced by various muscle attachments. It could also be used wherever guided bone regeneration is done. The steps are as follows:

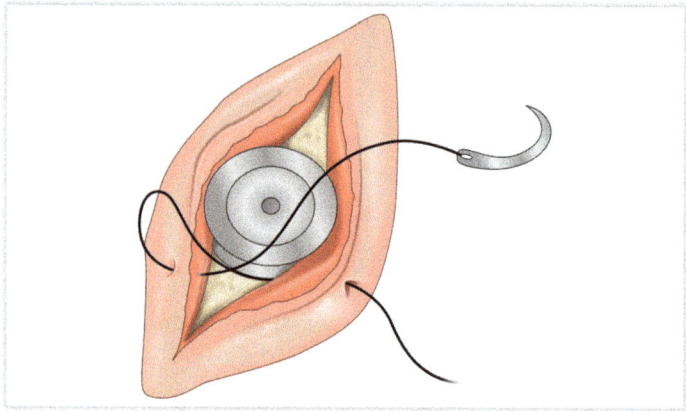

Fig. 14.8C: Needle repassed underneath contact point.

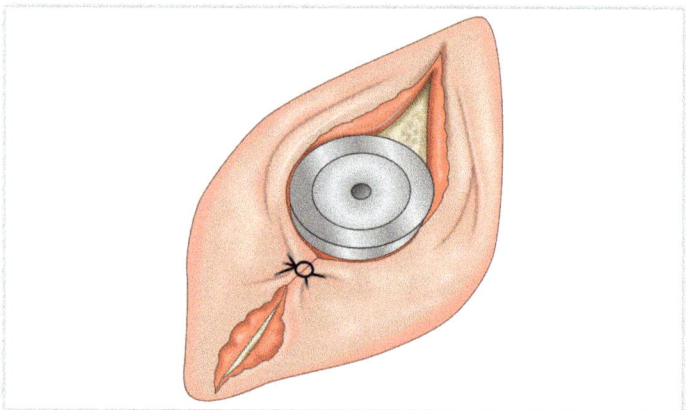

Fig. 14.8D: Knot tied on buccal surface.

1. Penetrate the buccal tissue flap from the outer surface 4 mm to 6 mm from the flap margin just above the level of the mucogingival margin with the tip of the needle in a coronal direction.
2. Pass the needle under the contact point.
3. Penetrate the inner side of the lingual flap 4–6 mm from the edge of the flap and then penetrate the outer side of the lingual flap 2–3 mm from the edge of the flap.
4. Pass it underneath the contact point and enter the inner surface of the buccal flap 2–3 mm from the flap edge and tie the knot on the buccal surface over the penetration of the needle (Figs. 14.10A to C).

Horizontal Mattress Suture Technique (Figs. 14.9A to D)

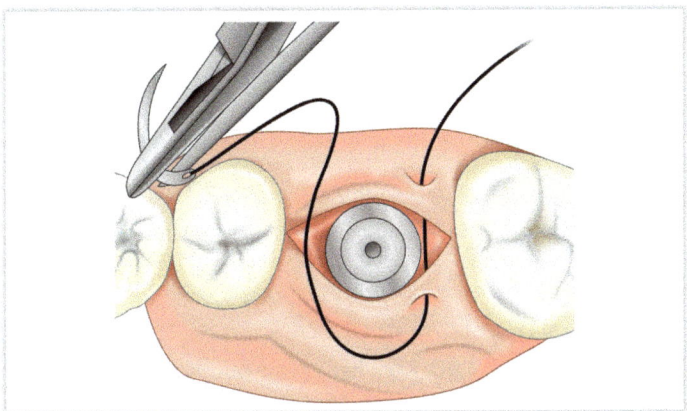

Fig. 14.9A: First entry of needle through outer surface of buccal flap, going underneath contact point and coming out through inner side of lingual flap.

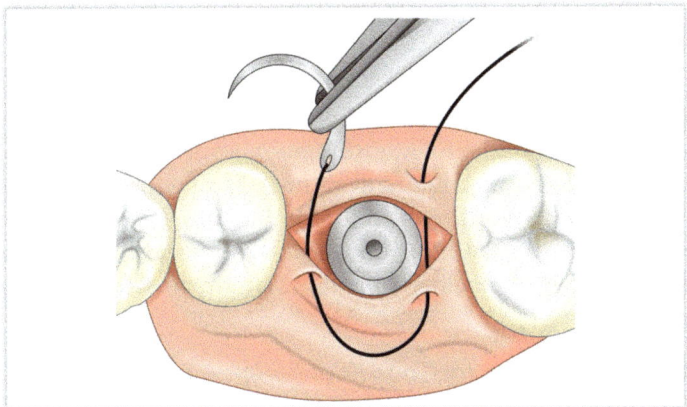

Fig. 14.9B: Needle entering from outer side of lingual flap.

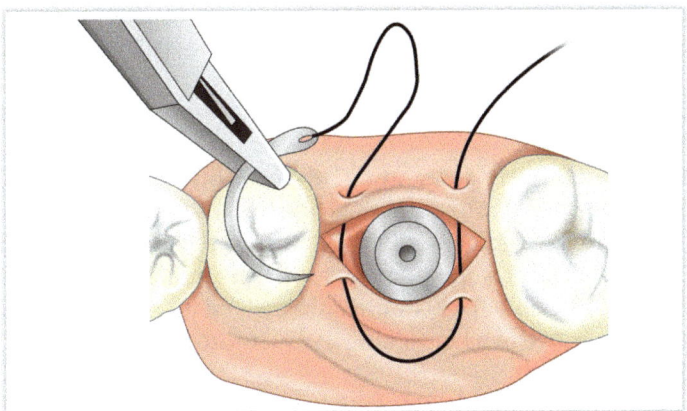

Fig. 14.9C: Needle passing under contact point and entering inner side on buccal flap.

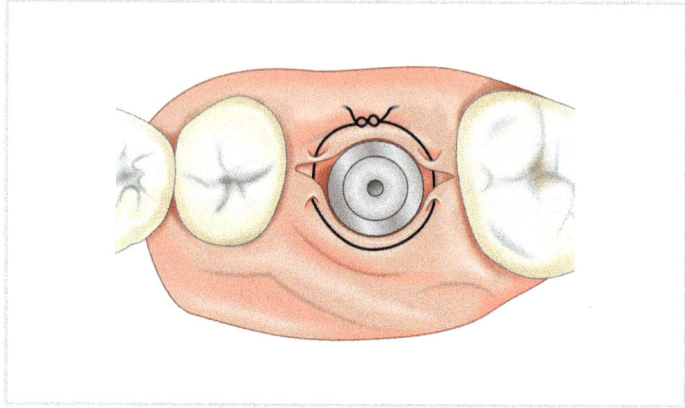

Fig. 14.9D: Knot tied on the buccal surface.

Surgical Knots

The type of knot to be employed to bring the wound edges together depends on the suture material used, and the amount of stress to be placed on the wound postoperatively. Multifilament sutures are generally easier to handle and tie than monofilament sutures. Knot tying requires meticulous attention and skill and therefore should be done slowly. The practitioner should consider the amount of tension being placed upon the incision line and should also take into consideration the postoperative edema that takes place.

Points to be Considered for Good Knot Tying

- In order to ensure a secure knot, the two ends of the suture must be pulled in different directions at an equal rate and with equal tension.
- The completed knot should be firm to prevent any slippage.
- The knot should be as small as possible and the ends of the knot should be cut 1 to 1.5 mm away from the knot.
- Excessive tension which may break the suture or cut through the tissues should be avoided.
- Never tie the suture too tightly. The idea is only to bring the edges of the incision together, not to traumatize the tissues.
- Trauma and strangulation due to increased tension will result in incision line opening with resultant healing with secondary intention.
- Traction at one end of the suture after the first loop should be maintained, otherwise there will be loosening of the suture knot.

Vertical Mattress Suture Technique (Figs. 14.10A to C)

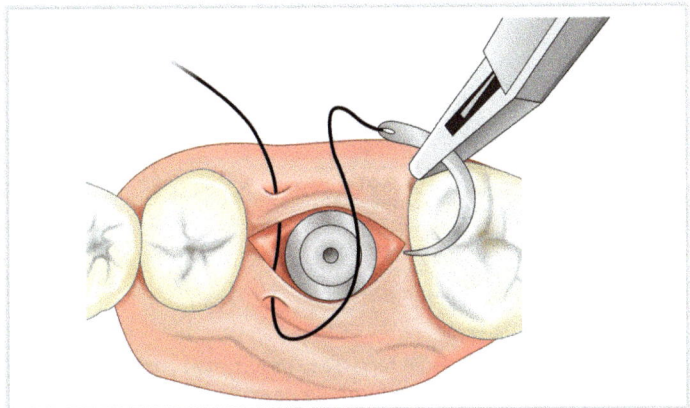

Fig. 14.10A: Needle entering at level of mucogingival junction 4–6 mm from flap margin.

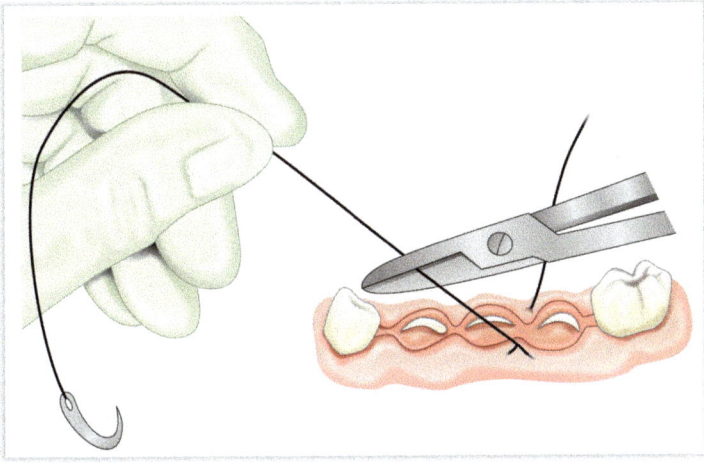

Fig. 14.10B: Needle passed underneath contact point through inner side of lingual flap and re-entered through outer side of lingual flap.

SURGEON'S KNOT

The surgeons knot is the most commonly used knot in implant surgery. Most intraoral sutures are tied with instrument tie.
- The suture is pulled through the tissues till the short tail of suture (2 inches long) remains (Fig. 14.11).

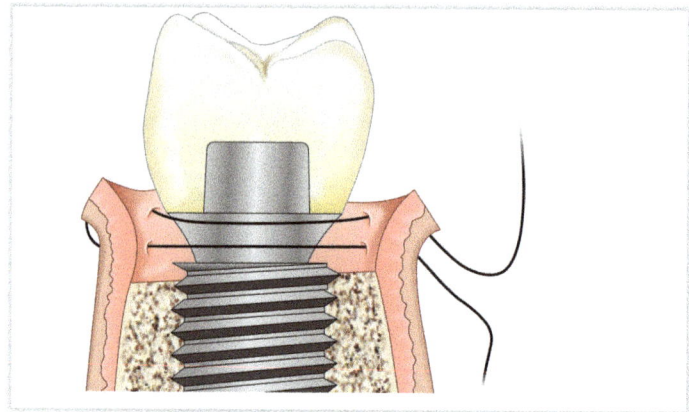

Fig. 14.10C: Needle repassed underneath contact point emerging out through inner side of buccal flap.

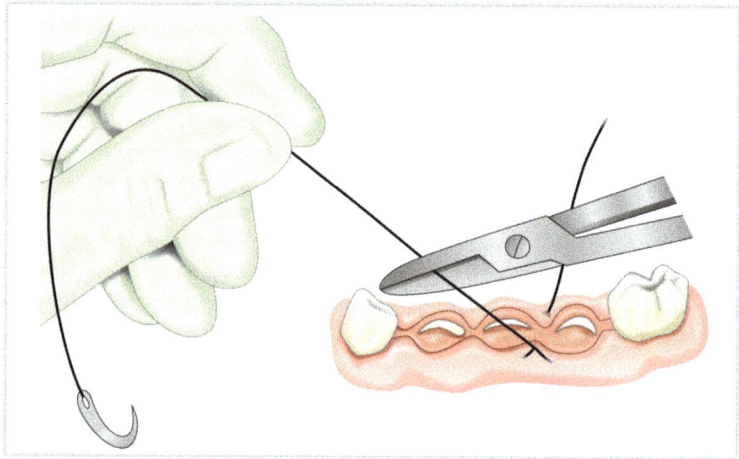

Fig. 14.11: Suture through tissue until short end of suture 2 inches long remain.

- Needle holder is held horizontally in right hand whilst left hand wraps the long end of the suture around needle holder twice in clockwise direction (Fig. 14.12).
- The needle holder then grasps short end of suture near its end and pulls to tighten the knot. The needle holder is not pulled until the knot is tied, otherwise this would lead to increasing the length of the short end. The double wrap helps in increasing the friction and keeps the knot tied until the second portion of the knot is tied (Fig. 14.13).
- The second knot is made by making a single wrap in the counter clockwise direction (Fig. 14.14).
- The third wrap is not compulsory but may be added in some cases to prevent unravelling.

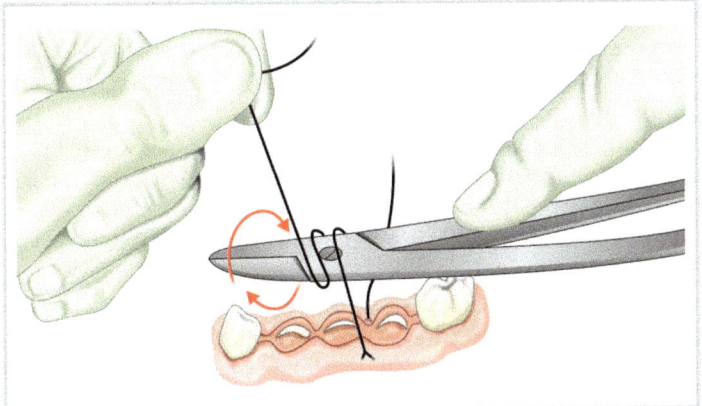

Fig. 14.12: Left hand wraps long end of suture twice in clockwise direction.

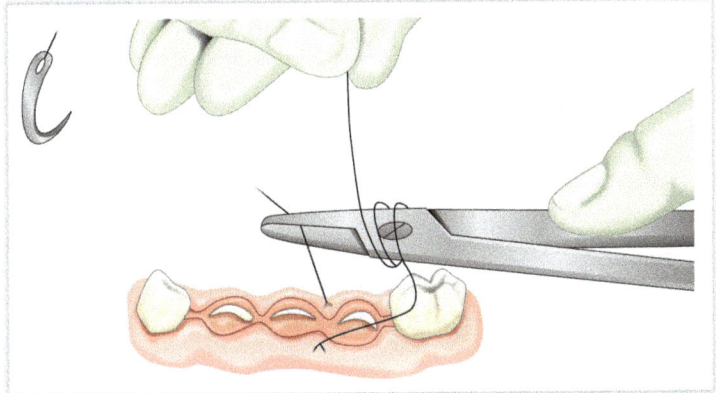

Fig. 14.13: Needle holder grasps short end of suture near its tail.

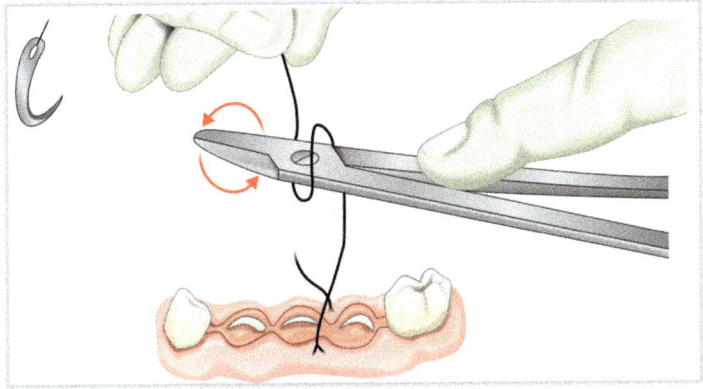

Fig. 14.14: Left hand making single warp in counter clockwise direction.

- When passing the needle through the mucosa always ensure that you pass it at right angles to the wound edge and not at an acute angle. This results in the smallest wound in the flap, thus reducing the chances of tearing through the flap, when the suture knot is tied.
- When suturing ensure that an adequate bite of tissue is taken from the incision line. The minimum tissue from the edge of the flap to the suture should be 3 mm.
- The knot should not be positioned over the incision line but to the side of it.
- Monofilament nylon suture knots have a tendency to loosen because of less friction generated by them. Multifilament braided suture knots because of their high coefficient of friction do not tend to slip and get united.
- The sutures generally should not be left in place for more than 7 to 10 days. After this period, they serve no useful purpose and may actually predisposes the wound to infection.
- The needle should always be first passed through the mobile (usually facial) tissue first and then through the attached lingual tissue.

RECOMMENDED READING

1. Silverstein LH. Principles of Dental Suturing: The Complete Guide to Surgical Closure, 1st Edition.

Chapter 15

Subepithelial Connective Tissue Grafting for Implant Aesthetics

The palate is the most preferred site for harvesting a subepithelial connective tissue graft. The subepithelial connective tissue graft contains collagen fibers and varying amounts of fatty and glandular tissues. The palatine artery should be protected as it is an extremely important anatomical structure. To reliably prevent damage to the posterior superior palatine artery (PSPA) the distal extension of the incision should end no further than the anterior surface of the first molar. Also care should be taken to see that the incision does not extend more than 10 mm from the sulcus of the maxillary molars. If placed about 2 mm from the sulcus, the initial incision can safely be extended 8 mm apically without fear of cutting the main branches of the superior alveolar artery. Because the working length of a no. 15 scalpel blade is roughly 8 mm, therefore it can help in safe harvesting of the connective tissue graft.

The single incision technique is the recommended method of choice for harvesting the subepithelial connective tissue graft. Studies have shown the single incision technique to be superior to other methods in terms of postoperative pain, healing and morbidity.[1-3] The main challenge is to achieve good healing of the donor site. If this is achieved postoperative complications are reduced.

The key to achieving this is to obtain a split thickness graft of uniform size. The initial incision should be made with the scalpel held perpendicular to the palatal surface to a depth of 1 to 1.5 mm in the superficial tissue layers and then successively parallel to the surface in the deeper tissue layers. It is also important to place the coronal incision for harvesting 1.5 mm apical to the first incision. This ensures that the flap rests not on the bone but on connective tissue which has a good source of blood supply and helps in primary wound closure.

It is better to harvest the graft with the periosteum because of better clinical handling while adapting to the recipient site or when the graft is sutured to the defect to prevent dehydration the graft should be immediately transferred to the receipt site or kept hydrated with normal saline. Parallel and crossed horizontal sling sutures are recommended to close the surgical site for primary wound healing. A postsurgical stent should be routinely used and is recommended for many reasons.

MODIFIED TUNNEL TECHNIQUE TO THICKEN MUCOSA AROUND IMPLANTS

The modified tunnel technique was developed by Zuhr et al. to ensure optimum nutrition to the connective tissue graft (CTG). A mucosal split thickness tunnel spanning several teeth is used to introduce the CTG graft. Patented tunneling knives are used to prevent flap perforation.[4]

A full thickness mucoperiosteal flap is elevated only in the papillary region. Blunt dissection of the papilla is done using papilla elevators.

Vertical double-crossed sutures are used to secure the graft. This suture immobilizes the flap and the graft in the coronal position and they compress the soft tissues against the implants and the roots of the adjacent teeth. Anatomical conditions around the implants are different from those around natural teeth. Peri-implant soft tissues have a poorer blood supply than the soft tissues around natural teeth because of the absence of periodontal ligament. Also the inter-proximal soft tissue height around implant is reduced. Therefore, when treating dehiscence around implants the defect will generally be classified as at least Millers Class III recession around natural teeth with the associated consequences of less coverage of dehiscence.

Therefore, although there will be an improvement complete coverage of the dehiscence defect should not be expected around implants[5] (Fig 15.1 to 15.9).

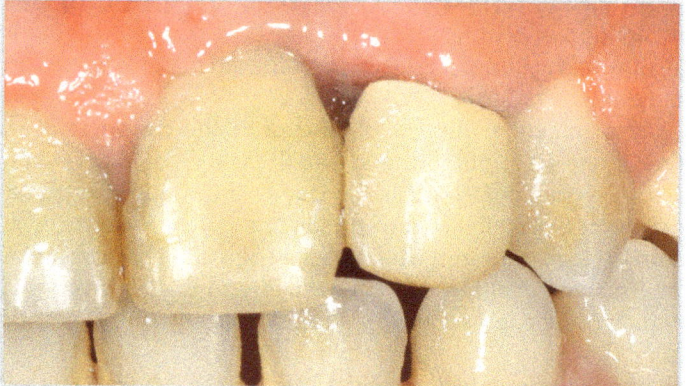

Fig 15.1: Although tissue have healed well after implant surgery and provisional restoration, there is a missing papilla and thin band of keratinized tissue.

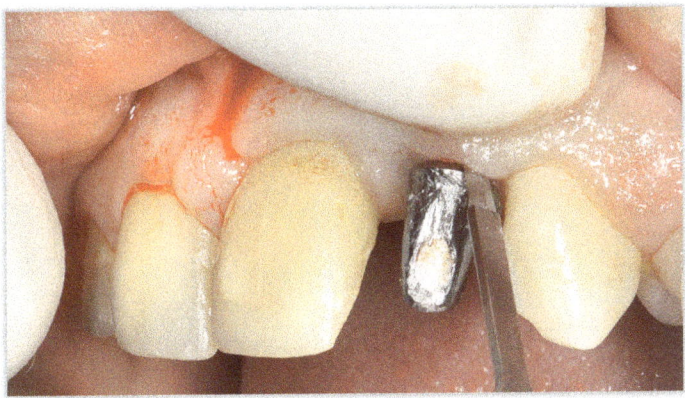

Fig. 15.2: Dissecting a partial-thickness flap with the aid of microsurgical scalpel blade.

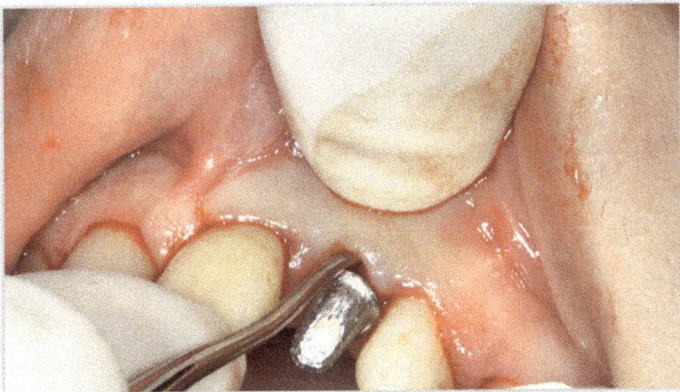

Fig. 15.3: Use of especially designed tunneling knives for preparation of partial thickness flaps according to the tunnel technique.

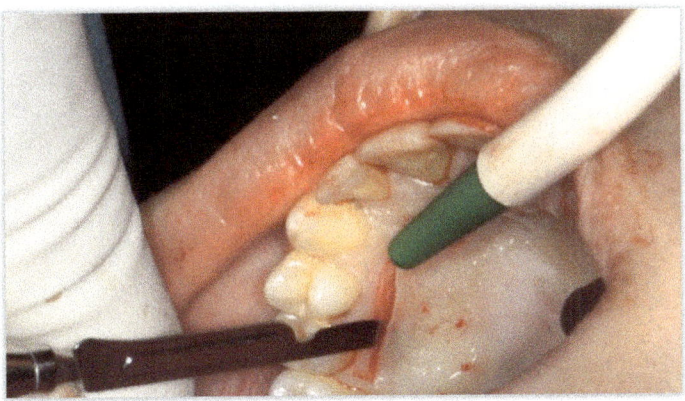

Fig. 15.4: The connective tissue graft (CTG) is next harvested from the palate.

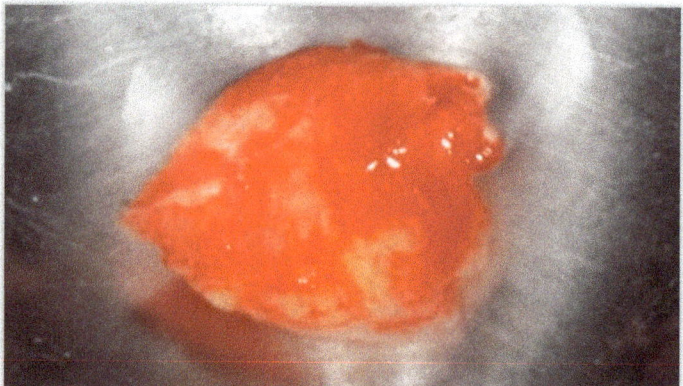

Fig. 15.5: Harvested CTG along with the periosteum.

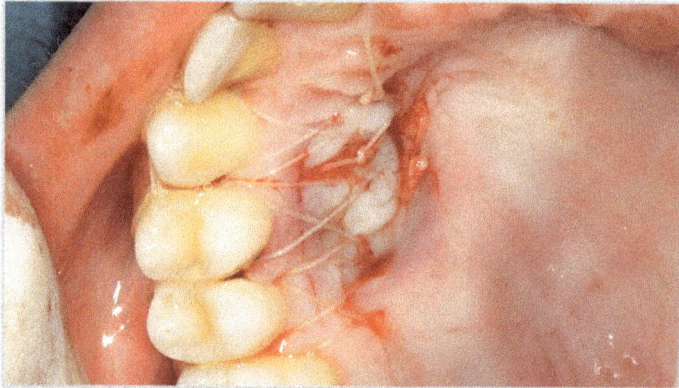

Fig. 15.6: Completion of the parallel and crossed horizontal sling sutures. The horizontal sling sutures have a compressing effect on the wound resulting in hemostasis and primary wound healing.

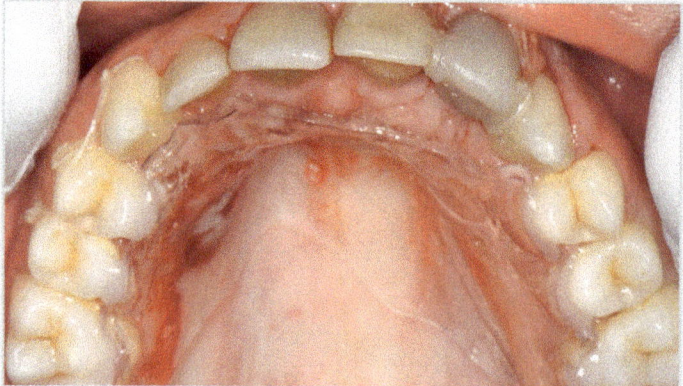

Fig. 15.7: Post-surgical palatal stent in place which helps in preventing bleeding by causing compression on the wound. It also keeps the patient comfortable by protecting the wound.

Subepithelial Connective Tissue Grafting for Implant Aesthetics

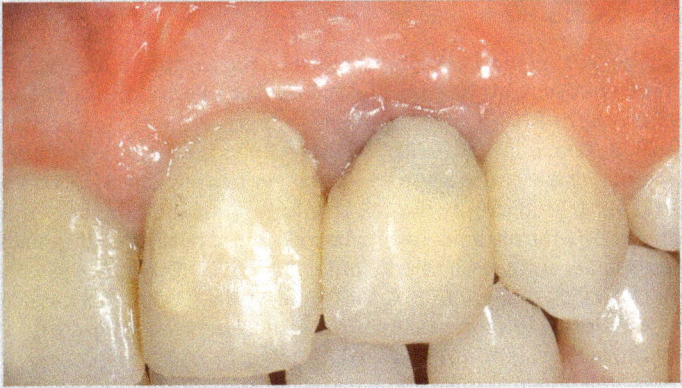

Fig. 15.8: Note the excellent thickening of peri-implant tissues after CTG grafting.

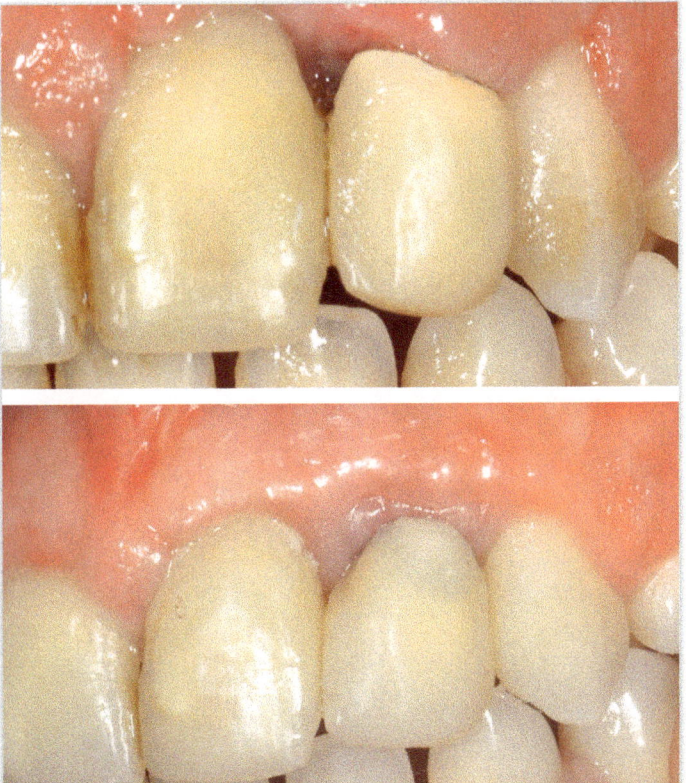

Fig. 15.9: Comparison of the soft tissues around the implant before CTG grafting and after CTG grafting. Note the increased band of thick keratinized tissue after grafting and regeneration of papilla.

REFERENCES

1. Hürzeler MB, Weng D. A single-incision technique to harvest subepithelial connective tissue grafts from the palate. Int J Periodontics Restorative Dent. 1999;19(3):279-87.
2. Wessel JR, Tatakis DN. Patient outcomes following subepithelial connective tissue graft and free gingival graft procedures. J Periodontol. 2008;79(3):425-30
3. Del Pizzo M, Modica F, Bethaz N, Priotto P, Romagnoli R. The connective tissue graft: a comparative clinical evaluation of wound healing at the palatal donor site. A preliminary study. J Clin Periodontol. 2002;29(9):848-54.
4. Zuhr O, Fickl S, Wachtel H, Bolz W, Hürzeler MB. Covering of gingival recessions with a modified microsurgical tunnel technique: case report. Int J Periodontics Restorative Dent. 2007;27(5):457-63.
5. Burkhardt R, Joss A, Lang NP. Soft tissue dehiscence coverage around endosseous implants: a prospective cohort study. Clin Oral Implants Res. 2008;19(5):451-7.

Chapter 16

Maintenance of Implant Rehabilitated Patients

Implant treatment has become a proven and very predictable treatment option. However, complications associated with implant treatment are not rare and unfortunately even with the most experienced and well-trained clinician cannot be completely prevented. Long-term complications related to biology and/or mechanics, also cannot be predicted. Therefore, implant dentistry implies the importance and compulsion of a strict aftercare protocol.

The difference between teeth and implant biologies suggest that dental implants are more susceptible to inflammation and bone loss in the presence of bacterial plaque accumulation as compared to natural teeth. Similar to teeth, clinical findings with failing implants include inflammation, pockets and bone loss. The bacterial flora responsible for periodontitis and peri-implantitis are also very similar.

Mucositis is an inflammation of soft tissues around an implant. It is similar to gingivitis in natural dentition. There is no loss of bone but there may be bleeding and inflamed soft tissue around the implant. The primary etiology is plaque biofilm. Mucositis-like gingivitis is preventable and reversible by proper oral hygiene measures and periodical aftercare treatment regimes. If mucositis is neglected, then it may proceed to peri-implantitis, bone destruction and even loss of osseointegration.

IMPORTANCE OF ORAL HYGIENE IN IMPLANT PATIENTS

Removal of supragingival plaque can significantly reduce the amount and composition of the subgingival microflora, which in turn can translate to decreased risk of peri-implantitis. The absence of adequate keratinized gingiva (less than 2 mm) has been shown to result in higher plaque accumulation and inflammation, however, the same studies have not been able to show bone loss regardless of the implant configuration. Therefore, in the absence of keratinized tissue more importance needs to be given to motivating patients to select products and procedures well suited to the needs and dexterity of the patients. Patients have confidence in the clinician to recommend reliable and proven oral care products. Patients should not only be shown on models but also in their mouths the correct method of brushing, also more importantly interdental and interimplant cleaning (Fig. 16.1). They must also be asked to demonstrate

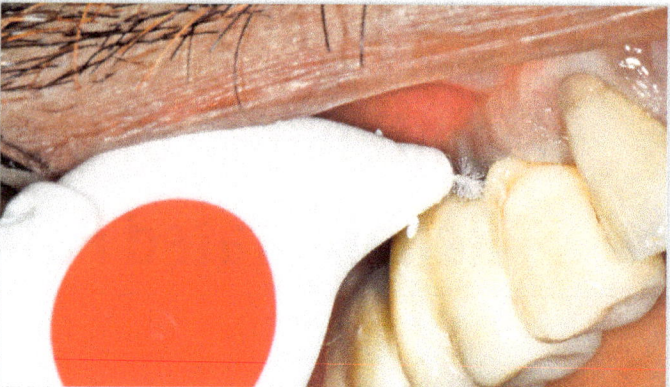

Fig. 16.1: Interdental brush use demonstrated.

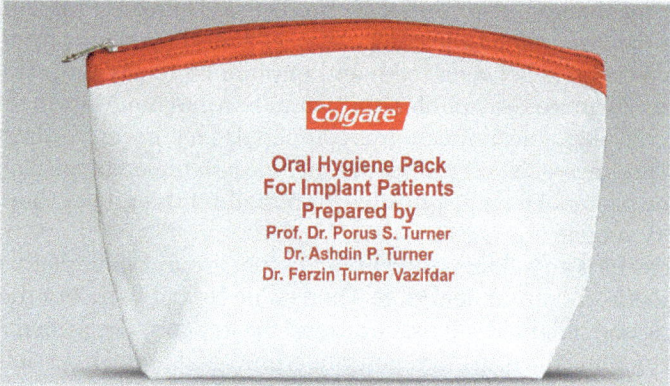

Fig. 16.2: Oral hygiene kit for implant patients.

the taught procedure on models to ascertain that they have understood and are able to follow the correct method of oral hygiene. The authors have developed an oral hygiene kit for the special use of implant patients which is given to the patients after explaining and making sure they have followed the instructions (Fig. 16.2). It consists of a soft tooth brush (Colgate Slim and Soft tooth brush, Colgate India), an antimicrobial toothpaste with substantive action[1,2] (Colgate Total Tooth Paste, Colgate India) and a chlorhexidine mouthwash[3] (Colgate Periogard, Colgate India). The giving away of the oral hygiene kit rather than just prescribing reinforces the importance of oral hygiene and further motivates the patients to strictly adhere to the protocol recommended. Chlorhexidine mouthwash (Periogard, Colgate India) is particularly useful for high-risk patients (Fig. 16.3), e.g. smokers, diabetic patients. Chlorhexidine gluconate has been shown to reduce plaque in the oral cavity and around the dental implants. In order to minimize staining it may be advised to be used with normal and interdental brushes instead of being used as a rinse. After a period of 15 days, implant patients can switch to a Cetylpyridinum mouth wash (Colgate Plax,

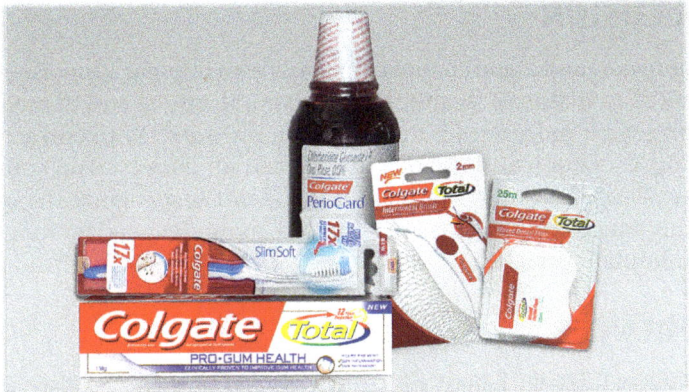

Fig. 16.3: Contents of oral hygiene kit for implant patients.

Colgate, India). Studies have shown that when proper oral hygiene is followed, then there is minimal inflammation of the peri-implant tissues.

SCHEDULE FOR MAINTENANCE OF IMPLANT PATIENTS

It is generally recommended that patients treated with implant retained prosthesis be seen every 4 months for evaluation. At every visit, oral hygiene instructions are reinforced and the patients dexterity in maintaining oral hygiene is checked. The peri-implant tissues around the implant are palpated gently and should not result in any bleeding or exudate nor should there be any pain. Probing depths maybe evaluated carefully and ideally should not be more than 4 mm with no bleeding.

ABUTMENT CONNECTION

Repeated chewing cycles, especially in bruxers may produce abutment loosening and creation of a gap between the implant and abutment which results in microbial colonization and inflammation. This complication can be prevented by attention to occlusal contacts and by adequately torquing the abutment screws. However, with the Ankylos system because of its conical morse taper implant abutment connection which produces a cold weld between the implant and abutment screw, loosening is extremely rare.

IMPORTANCE OF CESSATION OF TOBACCO HABITS

Nicotine and the toxic areosols in tobacco smoke directly influences the healing of oral tissues. The most relevant effects of smoking is a dose-dependent reduction of blood flow to tissues supplied by terminal vessels. Tobacco usage has also been found to reduce the immune defence of oral tissues.[4,5] Wound healing complications can occur in smokers, even if surgery is carefully planned and precisely executed.

CONCLUSION

Regular review and maintenance of patients with implant supported prosthesis is essential to maintain health, prevent complications and to measure one's own long-term success with the treatment provided. With correct treatment planning, execution and use of a time-tested implant system, complications are rare. Nevertheless, it is important that dentists recognize the importance of maintenance and patients are educated about the need for long-term care of their implant prosthesis.

REFERENCES

1. Ramberg P, Lindhe J, Botticelli D, Botticelli A. The effect of a triclosan dentifrice on mucositis in subjects with dental implants: a six-month clinical study. J Clin Dent. 2009;20(3):103-7
2. Sreenivasan PK, Vered Y, Zini A, Mann J, Kolog H, Steinberg D, et al. A 6-month study of the effects of 0.3% triclosan/copolymer dentifrice on dental implants. J Clin Periodontol. 2011;38(1):33-42.
3. Arweiler NB, Boehnke N, Sculean A, Hellwig E, Auschill TM. Differences in efficacy of two commercial 0.2% chlorhexidine mouth rinse solutions: a 4-day plaque regrowth study. J Clin Periodontol. 2006;33(5):334-9.
4. Johnson GK, Guthmiller JM. The impact of cigarette smoking on periodontal disease and treatment. Periodontol, 2000. 2007;44:178-94.
5. Palmer RM, Scott DA, Meekin TN, Poston RN, Odell EW, Wilson RF. Potential mechanisms of susceptibility to periodontitis in tobacco smokers. J Periodontal Res. 1999;34(7):363-9.

Index

Page numbers followed by *b* refer to box and *f* refer to figure.

A

Abutment 90*f*
   and prepared veneer 166*f*
   connection 207
   fitting within implant 37*f*
   position, accurate transfer of 150*f*
Acrylic resin, self-curing 144
Acteon
   intralift kit 71*f*
   sinus lift kit 76*f*
Adequate keratinized gingiva 205
Adjacent teeth, palatal surface of 183*f*
Aesthetic considerations 15
Algae-derived bone substitute 54
Allogenic bone 52, 53
   human 53
   irradiated 53
   solvent preserved 53
Alloplastic bone
   substitutes 53
   synthetic 53
Alloplastic grafting materials 53
Alloplasts 53
American Dental Association 4
Amoxycillin 23
Anesthesia 71
Ankylos 71
   balance sulcus 50*f*
   c/x implant 4
   implant 11*f*, 13*f*, 24, 34, 87, 98, 113, 139, 146*f*
      in place 62*f*
      placement of 26, 34
      shoulder of 26*f*
      site preparation 24
      system 21, 115*f*, 140, 174, 179
      template 31*f*
      with abutment 12*f*
   snap attachment 154
   syncone concept 134
   system 10, 12, 19, 31, 40, 69, 71, 207
Anodic oxidation surface 6
Antibiotic prophylaxis 23
Articulated study cast 17*f*
Atraumatic extraction 162*f*
Atrophic maxilla 95
Atrophic posterior maxilla, reconstruction of 69
Autogenous bone 53, 61, 66*f*, 129*f*
   mixed 56*f*

B

Beta-tricalcium phosphate 53
Bioactive glass 53
Biphosphonate therapy 19
Block bone graft 60*f*
   with delayed placement of implant 58
Blown down surgical stent 18*f*
Bluish membrane 75*f*
Bone
   allograft
      freeze dried 53
      mineralized freeze-dried 53
   biology 5
   contouring bur 29, 29*f*
   cruncher 64*f*
   destruction 205
   grafting 52
      with bio-OSS 85*f*
   growth in sinus cavity 100*f*
   harvested 53, 56*f*, 64*f*, 73*f*, 182*f*
   height measured 174*f*
   materials, natural components of 53
   position in 2
   regeneration 52, 54, 61

substitutes 53
   barrier membrane placed over 52*f*
   layered with 61
   to implant contact 6
Bony defect 55*f*
Bony window 85*f*
   removal of 84*f*
   replacing lateral 79*f*
Bridge, fixed 8
Buccal concavity 99*f*
Buccal contour, preservation of 171*f*
Buccal flap 191*f*, 193*f*, 196*f*
   outer part of 189*f*
Buccal plate of bone 167
Buccal wall 164*f*, 170*f*
   grafting of 170*f*
Butt joint implant abutment 13*f*

C

Calcium sulphate 53
Calibrated caliper 16*f*
Canine
   regions 47*f*
   upper right 148*f*
   vertical fracture of 2*f*
Capability of ankylos 134
Cast
   duplicate upper 141*f*
   with gingival mask 49*f*
Cemented porcelain-fused-to-metal splinted crowns 93*f*
Ceramic crowns 63*f*, 67*f*
Ceramo-metal bridge cemented 160*f*
Cerasorb 53
Cervical threads 25*f*
Chlorhexidine 23*f*, 90
   gluconate oral rinse 137
   mouthwash 206
Cingulum for minicrown preparation 44*f*
Clindamycin 23, 80
Clonazepam 23
Closed mouth impression, posts placed for 143*f*
Collagen membrane 62*f*, 79*f*
Columnar epithelial cells 95

Complete denture
   stabilization 154
   supported 146*f*
   upper 145*f*
Complete flap reflection 29*f*
Complete maxillary denture 12*f*
   stability of 139
Complete overdenture supported by syncone abutments 9*f*
Condense bone 148*f*
Cone beam computed tomography 19, 74
Conical reamer flushed with bone crest 33*f*
Conical reamer
   salient features of 33
   use of 36*f*, 141*f*
Connective tissue graft 200, 201*f*
Cord
   completed packing of 42*f*
   removal of 42*f*
Crestal bone 13*f*
   levels, excellent 173*f*
   loss 108, 109
   preservation of 108
Crestal incision 72*f*, 147, 183*f*
   with median tissue bridge intact 136*f*
Crestal sinus floor elevation 95
Crown 58*f*
   on maxillary left canine 9*f*
   temporarily cemented, composite 165*f*

D

Dental implants, types of 2
Dentsply implants 10, 12, 19
Dentsply sirona implant 1, 4, 6, 21, 71, 87
Denture
   final polished surface of 157*f*
   in mouth in centric occlusion 152*f*
   intaglio surface of 152*f*, 157*f*
   over 8
   polished surface of 152*f*
De-proteinized bovine bone material 169
Diclofenac 23
Die stone poured 49*f*

E

Endodontic file 17*f*
Endosseous implant 4, 4*f*
Esthetics, high end 161
Extraction sockets 108*b*

F

Facebow transfer 160*f*
Figure of eight suture, closing of wound with 170*f*
Fine needle holder 188*f*
Flap
   and suturing 86*f*
   dissecting partial-thickness 201*f*
Flapless procedure 109
Floor of sinus 70*f*
Fracture
   central incisor 116
   floor of sinus 102*f*
   of lateral incisor, horizontal 1*f*
   of weak lateral incisor abutment 8*f*
   root, atraumatic luxation of 117*f*
   sinus floor 99*f*

G

Gingiva, healing of 50*f*
Gingival
   health 40
      working time 41
   margin, free 114*f*, 126*f*
   mask
      being poured 48*f*
      in place 48*f*
   retraction 41
      cord placed 132*f*
Gold caps 138*f*
Grafted sinus cavity, infection of 80
Granulation tissue, formation of 80
Green-stick fracture 148*f*
Gutta-percha 136*f*

H

Hard and soft tissues, maintenance of 153*f*
Healing after 3 weeks 145*f*
Hemostat 188*f*
Hydrodynamic piezoelectric internal sinus floor elevation 95
Hydroxyl apatite 24

I

Implant 142*f*
   aesthetics 121
      subepithelial connective tissue grafting for 199
   after placement, two 177*f*
   analogs 49*f*
      attachment to 143*f*
   angulations 136*f*
   before prosthetic rehabilitation 9*f*
   coronal part of 65*f*
   delayed loading of 146
   direct impression recording position of 160*f*
   exposure of 184*f*
   final placement of 114*f*
   grafting and placement of 104*f*
   healing 5
   in grafted bone, placement of 57*f*
   in place immediately after grafting 100*f*
   in upper and lower jaw, placement of 145*f*
   level impression technique 49*f*
   maintenance of 205, 207
   motorized insertion of 36*f*
   number 19
   osteotomies, position of 136*f*
   part of 65*f*
   placement 13*f*, 54, 55*f*, 62*f*, 88*f*, 89*f*, 108, 170*f*, 174
      advantages of immediate 108*b*
      complications after 179
      grafting and 100*f*
   size 19
   spacing 19
   subcrestal placement of 137*f*
   submerged 35
   subperiosteal 3, 3*f*
   supported fixed bridge 8*f*
   supported prosthesis
      fixed 14*f*
      impression making for 40, 45

surgery, basic 21
three-dimensional placement of 126f
tissue interphase 5
to bone contact 87
transferring orientation of 49f
treatment 205
uncovering of 38f, 171f
width of 60f
with forceps, removal of 181f
with placement heads exhibiting 142f
Implantation
immediate 167
prerequisites for immediate 110b
Implantology 1
Implant-retained
fixed bridges 8
overdentures 10
Impression
making, repositioning technique of 50f
material
accurate 40
after removal 181f
syringing of 41
removal of 47f
technique 41
Incision 83f
line opening 80
up to adjacent teeth 27f
Incisors, central 47f
Initial osteotomy, positioning of 168f
Instrumentation, quality of 4
Interdental papilla, spontaneous regeneration of 58
Interrupted suture technique 189
modified 191
Intralift kit 96f, 99f
Intraoral
occlusal view 92f
of failed implant 183f
of fractured tooth 111f
view, preoperative 82f, 140f, 167f
Intrasulcular incisions 109

J

Jaw relation recorded 151f

K

Keratinized tissue, thin band of 200f
Knot tied on buccal
side 190f
surface 192f, 194f

L

Lindemann drill 30f, 35, 69
sequential use of 162f
Lingual flap 190f, 191f, 193f
mobilization of 28f
Lithium disilicate crowns after cementation 67f
Luxated root, removal of 117f
Luxator, use of 112f, 168f

M

Mandibular nerve, anterior loop of 174
Mattress suture technique
horizontal 191, 193
vertical 191, 195
Maxilla, anterior 108
Maxillary
overdentures 10
sinus, grafting of 69
Mayo tray 23f
Membrane
after removal of bony window 77f
elevation 84f
on right side 86f
platelet rich fibrin 105
Mental foramen
coronal to inferior alveolar canal 176f
identification of 175f
Mesial and distal surface 112f
Microsurgical blades, periotomes 121
Midcrestal incision 27f
Monofilament nylon 186
Mucogingival junction, level of 195f
Mucoperiosteal flaps, reflection of 26
Mucositis 205
Mucositis-like gingivitis 205

N

Nasal opine with chisel 182f
Nasal spine 56, 129f

Nicotine 207
Noble biocare implants 6
Noble implant system 4
Non-eugenol temporary
 cement 115*f*, 120*f*
Non-salvageable upper right central
 incisor 116*f*

O

Open tray
 impression posts in place 149*f*
 technique 46*f*
Optimal bone quality 121
Oral anxiolytic agents 23
Oral hygiene
 in implant patients 205
 kit
  contents of 207*f*
  for implant patients 206*f*
Orthopantomogram, preoperative 111*f*
Orthopantomography 7
Osseointegration 2, 6
 loss of 205
Osteoblast deposition 26*f*
Osteophylic phase 5
Osteotome 70*f*
 to condense bone 141*f*
 use of 36*f*, 141*f*
Osteotome-mediated sinus floor
 elevation 95
Osteotomy 69, 71, 109, 126
 and drill in posterior, anterior 31*f*
 and implant placement 5
 in compromised bone 35
 initial 30*f*
 preparation of 29, 118*f*
 site 184
 with conical reamer 32*f*

P

Palatal alveolar bone 64*f*
Palatal cortical bone 118*f*
Palatal crest 169*f*
Palatine artery, posterior superior 199
Panoramic radiograph,
 postoperative 139*f*

Papilla
 elevator reflecting marginal
  tissues 28*f*
 elevator, discoid-shaped
  semi-sharp 28*f*
 lack of 132*f*
 missing 200*f*
 regeneration of 203*f*
 spontaneous regeneration of 59*f*
Paracetamol 23
Partial denture
 fixed 59*f*, 61, 156*f*
 with provisional removable 16*f*
 without provisional removable 15*f*
Partial thickness flaps, preparation
 of 201*f*
Particulate mineral bovine bone 123*f*
Peri-implant tissues 203*f*
 healthy 58
Peri-implantitis 180*f*, 182*f*, 205
Periodontal fibers 112*f*
 severe 111
Periosteal blood, fresh 74*f*
Periosteum 109, 202*f*
Piezosurgery 59
Piezotome 96*f*
Pilot drill 30
Plasma spraying 24
Platelet-derived growth factors 104
Plus clavulanic acid 23
Polyglactin 186
Polyglycolic acid 187
Porcelain fused-to-metal crowns
 splinted 91*f*, 92*f*
Porcelain laminate veneer 165*f*
Post-surgical palatal stent 202*f*
Prosthesis
 cemented in patient's mouth, fixed
  49*f*
 replacing, fixed 98
Prosthodontics, quality of 4
Provisional restoration 127*f*, 108*b*, 132*f*

R

Reamer with nentwig instrument 164*f*
Resorbable collagen membrane 66*f*, 78*f*
Restoration, fixed 158

Retraction cord 58f
Root forcep, rotational movements of 117f
Root fracture, vertical 55f

S

Scalpel blade, aid of microsurgical 201f
Schneiderian membrane 76
Scissors 187
Sculpt tissues 172f
Silicone sleeve
    covering lamella 155f
    removal of 157f
Simple interrupted suture technique 189
Simultaneous impression technique 51f
Single tooth restorations 8, 12
Sinus
    cavity
        access window to 74
        grafting 79f
        lateral wall of 73f
    curette 77f
    floor 70f
    grafting 69, 78, 95
    membrane 76, 77f
        elevation curettes 77f
        elevation of 76
        management of perforation of 76
    tenting 70f
    with osteotomes, lifting 69
    surgery
        kit 75
        patients, maintenance of 90
Sling sutures 202f
Snap attachment
    abutments 154
    region of 156f
Socket
    grafting before flap reflection 130f
    palatal wall of 164f
Soft denture liner during interim period 150f
Soft tissue
    around implant 203f
    infiltration, prevent 62f
    management 121
    recession 184f
Stabilized collagen membrane 56f
Stay suture in place 73f

Stent with radiographic markers 18f
Sticky bone 105f
    preparation of 105f
Straumann implant system 4
Sulcus
    formers in place 156f
    removal of 50f
Supragingival plaque, removal of 205
Surgeon's knot 195
Surgical knots 194
Surgical procedure 35, 81, 135
Surgical protocol 21
Surgical stent, step in preparation of 14f
Surgical suction unit 21f
Surgical technique 69, 71, 97
Surgical torque control motor 22f
Suture scissor 189f
Suturing instruments 187
Suturing techniques 189
Suturing, principles of 186
Syncone abutments 11f, 137f
    dentsply implants 10
    paralleled 144f
Syncone caps 11f, 138f, 145f
    in place on abutments 144f
    with cast metal framework 12f
Syncone gold caps cemented to metal framework 151f
Syncone treatment concept 139

T

Tacking pins 56f
Tapping thread 34
Temporary crown 115f
    cemented 115f
    placed 177f
Thicken mucosa around implants 200
Tissue forceps 187
Tissue-holding forcep, delicate 188f
Tobacco habits, cessation of 207
Toxic areosols 207
Trabecular bone 25f
Transgingival healing 34
    with aid of sulcus former 35f
    with gingival formers 106f
Transosseous implant 3, 3f
Tray technique, combination of open and closed 46f

Treatment plan 7, 135, 140
Trephine burs 64*f*
Tricalcium phosphates 53
Tunnel technique 201*f*
  modified 200*f*

U

Ustomed kit 59

V

Valsalva's maneuver 97
Versatility 4
Vertical double-crossed sutures 200

W

Wel-documented cell occlusive 65
Window outline, drilling of 83*f*

Wound healing
  excellent 171
  hemostasis and primary 202*f*
  surgical 5

X

Xenogenic bone 52, 53
  grafts
    chemically treated 54
    thermally treated 54

Z

Zirconia
  abutment 165*f*
  all ceramic crowns 178*f*
  crown 58
  implants 4

EU GSPR Authorised Reprsentative
Logos Europe, 9 rue Nicolas Poussin
1700, La Rochelle, France
Phone: +33 (0) 6 67 93 73 78
E-mail: contact@logoseurope.eu

www.ingramcontent.com/pod-product-compliance
Ingram Content Group UK Ltd.
Pitfield, Milton Keynes, MK11 3LW, UK
UKHW050427150426
5217IPUK00019B/1274